WELLNESS—
The Inside Story

JULIA SWARNER Dr. P.H.

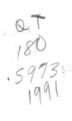

Pacific Press Publishing Association
Boise, Idaho
Oshawa, Ontario, Canada

Edited by Marvin Moore
Designed by Tim Larson
Cover photo by The Image Bank®/John P. Kelly
Typeset in 10/12 Century Schoolbook

Library of Congress Cataloging-in-Publication Data

Swarner, Julia, 1940-
    Wellness—the inside story: improving the quality of your life /
Julia Swarner.
        p.   cm.
    ISBN 0-8163-0935-3 (pbk.)
    1. Nutrition. 2. Reducing. 3. Self-care, Health. I. Title.
RA784.S89 1991   90-62278
613.2—dc20   CIP

91 92 93 94 95 • 5 4 3 2 1

Contents

To my husband,
O. Ward Swarner, M.D.,
and my children, Stephanie, Scott, and Stephen,
with love.

Introduction

Something exciting is happening across America. A war is being waged on the number-one killer of its people, and the enemy is in retreat. Twenty years ago *more than half* of all American deaths were from coronary heart disease. Today 36 percent are. The most powerful weapons in this fight have not come from the intensive care unit or even the skilled surgeon's hand, but from a change in lifestyle freely chosen by the American people.

But we've just scratched the surface! We now know that *five* of the top ten causes of death in the United States are directly related to nutrition. What we eat profoundly affects the length and quality of our lives. Applying these discoveries could have an enormous impact! But no lives will be longer or more free of pain or more filled with joy until people know what changes are needed and make them.

This book was written to communicate to the concerned and wise citizen new knowledge from nutrition research and how it can change the quality and length of life.

Chapter 1

The cholesterol dilemma

I didn't know his name, but I liked him. A gray-haired man in his sixties, he walked the same route I jogged every morning. His smile was so open and his "Good morning" so friendly. Then one day I missed him. Maybe I was a little later than usual, I thought. That afternoon a neighbor stopped me and asked, "Did you know Joe Watson? He walked along here every morning when you do. He died this morning."

"Oh, no! Heart attack?"

"Yes."

The next day our daughter Stephanie came home from summer camp, and I told her about it. "Yes, I knew him," she cried. "I can't believe it! Oh, I feel so sorry for his wife."

"What ever-widening circles of grief and pain derive from the loss of a single life," I thought as Stephanie busied herself making banana bread for Mrs. Watson. Yet scenes like this will be enacted over half a million times this year across America as coronary heart disease continues to take its toll.

It is not surprising that I was able to guess the cause of Mr. Watson's death, because coronary heart disease is the leading killer in the United States. My second guess would have been stroke. The underlying cause of both heart attack and stroke is often the same—atherosclerosis. If an artery supplying the heart muscle is completely blocked, a heart attack results. If an artery supplying part of the brain becomes clogged, the person has a stroke. Heart attacks and strokes taken together account for *half* of all the deaths in America. The picture is very different in developing countries. Even in the United States, death from coronary heart disease is not common before middle age, but then it reaches almost epidemic proportions, especially in males over forty-five. After menopause, American women have just as many heart attacks and even more strokes than do men of the same age.

Since atherosclerosis is so deadly, can anything be done to fight it? Absolutely! Progress against this killer is being made. In fact, the American death rate from coronary heart disease is a third lower now than it was twenty years ago.

Part of this decrease is due to advances in medical treatment, such as new drugs to control high blood pressure and improved surgical procedures such as the coronary bypass and balloon angioplasty. But *most* of the drop in heart disease deaths is due to *lifestyle changes*, like stopping smoking and healthier eating and exercise habits. It is now clear that atherosclerosis is often closely related to lifestyle, and that there are many ways to reduce the risk of coronary heart disease. To understand them, it is necessary to know something about how atherosclerosis develops.

The beginnings

Mr. Watson's heart attack happened without warning. Yet it didn't "just happen." Years ago—probably during his childhood—the stage was silently being set within his blood vessels. Three layers compose the walls of the arteries, and the innermost coat is the site where atherosclerosis begins. The first sign is just a streak of fat embedded in this layer. Gradually, more fatty material is deposited. A plaque begins to form, and at first it is soft and mushy and made of the same fatty substances as are floating in the blood.

What causes this process to start, we do not know. An injury to the artery wall, viruses, inherited factors—all are possibilities. These changes are seen in most males living in affluent countries early in life, during childhood. As the plaque continues to develop, more connective tissue forms and the artery wall becomes stiff. Eventually, calcium is also deposited in the plaque, and the artery becomes inflexible at that site. As more and more fatty material builds up in the plaque, the opening within the artery becomes smaller and smaller till eventually it is blocked completely.

Autopsies on American soldiers killed during the Korean and Vietnamese wars showed that *most* of them, young men in their late teens and early twenties, had already developed fibrous plaques. Since we know that stress fosters atherosclerosis, we might have concluded that the stressful war conditions were at fault—except for the fact that autopsies on enemy Oriental soldiers didn't reveal such plaques.

Lipids in the blood

Since the early stages of atherosclerosis are silent and no symptoms are present, is there any way to know what is happening? Actually, there are several ways. One way is to inject a dye into the bloodstream and then take X-rays of the coronary arteries. Since this must be done in a hospital and it involves some risk and is expensive, another method is more popular. This test, often done as a part of a routine physical exam, simply measures the amount of fatty substances in the blood. These fatty substances are called *lipids*. There are many types of lipids in the blood, and too much of one or more of them is a red flag warning of potential plaque formation. Just as repeatedly pouring grease down a drain may eventually cause it to become clogged, so high levels of blood lipids are likely to result in narrowing of the arteries.

All fats are lipids, but not all lipids are fats.

Cholesterol is an example of a lipid that is not a fat. Cholesterol is the blood lipid most often measured to assess a person's risk of developing coronary heart disease. It has been so maligned that one might wonder why such a treacherous compound is even in the body. Actually, cholesterol is an important component of the brain, nerves, and cell membranes, and is needed for making vitamin D, bile salts, and several hormones, including the sex hormones. But even though cholesterol is essential to life, abnormally high levels in the blood have been strongly correlated with an increased risk of coronary heart disease.

So if your dad, brother, and Uncle Harry all had heart attacks and your mother died of a stroke, you had better run— not walk—to your physician and have your blood cholesterol level measured. Even if atherosclerosis doesn't run in your family, knowing your blood cholesterol level is important.

How much is too much? Values considered normal vary somewhat from one laboratory to another, but here at Loma Linda University Medical Center we consider 150-220 milligrams percent to be the normal range. Remember, though, that normal ranges have been set according to the levels seen among *apparently* healthy Americans. Since half of all Americans are dying of causes related to atherosclerosis, it is believed that keeping the blood cholesterol level below 200 milligrams percent (200 milligrams of cholesterol per 100 millilters of blood) is best.

Three major risk factors

A high blood cholesterol level is one of the three primary risk factors known to increase a person's chances of developing coronary heart disease. The other two are high blood pressure (hypertension) and cigarette smoking. These three risk factors are interrelated. If a person has one of them his chance of developing atherosclerosis is twice what it would be in a person who has none of them. Two factors triple the risk, and if all three are present the risk is ten times greater!

Of these three primary risk factors, a high blood cholesterol level seems to be the most important, because the effects of cigarette smoking and high blood pressure are weakened if blood cholesterol levels are not also elevated.

Three Major Risk Factors for Coronary Heart Disease	
1. High Blood Pressure	Normal: 120/80 Hypertensive: above 140/90
2. Cigarette Smoking	
3. High Blood Cholesterol	Over 200 milligrams percent (mg in 100 milliliters of blood)

Years of research have shown beyond any doubt that keeping the level of blood cholesterol below 200 milligrams percent of blood protects against atherosclerosis. Just a 1 percent decrease in blood cholesterol levels results in a 2 percent decrease in the incidence of heart attack. A 10 percent reduction in blood cholesterol (say from 250 to 225) cuts a person's chance of having a heart attack by one-fifth, and a 25 percent drop cuts the risk in half. Obviously, lowering your blood cholesterol level can be very worthwhile. It can even *reverse* existing plaques! That is why medical science has put forth such a great deal of effort to identify the lifestyle factors that lower blood cholesterol levels.

Altering blood cholesterol levels

For scientists wanting to understand the relationship between lifestyle and cholesterol, one of the most obvious places to start looking seemed to be the relationship between the amount of cholesterol a person ate and the amount of cholesterol in his or her blood. It was discovered that an adult's body can make all the cholesterol it needs, even when the diet is cholesterol free. On the other hand, eating large amounts of cholesterol does increase blood cholesterol levels in many people. The average American eats about 600 milligrams of cholesterol a day. The American Heart Association recommends limiting daily intake of cholesterol to no more than 300 milligrams.

What foods contain cholesterol? Cholesterol is an animal product, so it is found only in foods of animal origin. Since plants can't make cholesterol, fruits, grains, nuts, and vegetables contain none at all. A quick look at the chart on page 14 will show that organ meats and egg yolk are particularly high in cholesterol. It is important to realize that cholesterol is in the fat, so animal products such as skim milk and egg whites will be virtually cholesterol free. Low-fat animal products such as lean meats, skim milk cheeses, low-fat milk, low-fat cottage cheese, etc., will still contain some cholesterol, but much will have been removed along with the fat.

Fat facts. Further investigation led to a surprising discovery: A diet high in saturated fat has an even more powerful

Cholesterol Content of Selected Foods

Cholesterol is a normal constituent of the blood and tissues. The cholesterol in the diet is only one of many factors that influences the amount of cholesterol in the blood. The National Institute of Health recommends decreasing cholesterol intake to 250-300 mg per day for the prevention of coronary heart disease.

Cholesterol is not present in plant foods, such as fruits, vegetables, grains, nuts, and legumes. The following list indicates the approximate amounts of cholesterol found in some foods.

FOOD*	AMOUNT	CHOLESTEROL (MG)
Meat and Eggs		
Brains	3 oz.	2110
Kidney	3 oz.	398
Liver	3 oz.	319
Egg yolk	1	225
Veal	3 oz.	96
Beef	3 oz.	75
Pork	3 oz.	75
Chicken	3 oz.	68
Egg white	1	0
Fish and Seafood		
Shrimp	3 oz.	128
Crab	3 oz.	86
Lobster (meat only)	3 oz.	72
Salmon, canned	3 oz.	35
Dairy Products		
Cheese, cheddar	3 oz.	84
Ice cream (regular)	1 cup	54
Butter	1 tbsp.	35
Milk, whole	1 cup	34
Milk, low-fat	1 cup	22
Milk, nonfat	1 cup	5
Plant Products		
Fruits		0
Vegetables		0
Grains and cereals		0
Nuts		0
Legumes		0

*Meat values are for cooked form.

Information based on "Composition of Foods," Agriculture Handbook no. 8, U.S. Department of Agriculture, Washington, D.C., 1975.

effect on raising the blood cholesterol level than a diet high in cholesterol. Even more astonishing was the finding that eating *unsaturated* fats actually *lowered* blood cholesterol levels! However, a given amount of saturated fat raised blood cholesterol levels approximately twice as much as the same amount of unsaturated fat lowered them. Obviously, the *type* of fat in the diet is profoundly important.

All sorts of foods are now advertised as being "cholesterol free," low in saturated fat, or high in unsaturated fat. However, the consumer must be armed with a certain amount of knowledge to avoid being misled. For example, since cholesterol is an animal product, advertising that peanut butter is cholesterol free is certainly true, but it would be more helpful if the label stated the *type* of fat present. Since they are made from vegetable fats, nondairy creamers do not contain cholesterol, but many are high in saturated fat.

Actually, it is easy to choose wisely if you understand a few guidelines. Saturated fats (the bad guys) are usually solid at room temperature. Unsaturated fats (the good guys) are usually liquid at room temperature. Almost all fats of animal origin are saturated. Vegetable fats that have been hardened by hydrogenation, as in the case of stick margarines and solid shortenings, are also saturated. Beef fat and lard are especially highly saturated. Chicken fat is less saturated and fish oils are even more unsaturated.

Almost all fats of vegetable origin are unsaturated. Exceptions to this rule are coconut and palm oils. At first this fact may seem unimportant, since Americans do not traditionally use coconut and palm oil in cooking. However, a large number of commercially available products contain these fats. Two examples are certain imitation sour creams and some nondairy creamers. Reading food labels can be very enlightening. The ingredients are listed in descending order, according to the amount present in the product. The first ingredient listed is present in the largest amounts.

Most Americans eat twice as much saturated fat as unsaturated fat, whereas the opposite should be true. The American Heart Association recommends that 30 percent or less of the daily caloric intake come from fat, and of the fat calories, no more than one-third should be from saturated fat. The average American gets about 40 percent of his calories as fat. The Fats of Life chart that begins on page 74 will help you to judge your own diet. Some of the most important facts you need to know about saturated and unsaturated fats are mentioned below:

Saturated fats	*Unsaturated fats*
• Solid at room temperature	• Liquid at room temperature
• Include most animal fats, hydrogenated vegetable fats	• Include most vegetable fats
• Examples: lard, beef fat, butter	• Example: vegetable oils
• Raise blood cholesterol	• Lower blood cholesterol

Defeating cholesterol

How does all this translate into food? Is it even possible to "eat to your heart's content" without taking all the joy out of life? Yes, it really is, but don't try to revolutionize your diet all at once. Tastes change slowly, but they do change, and the time will come when you will wonder why you were ever wedded to the typical American diet that is so high in saturated animal fat.

Start by making small changes. You can still eat the things you love. Just eat less of your high-fat favorites, or modify the way they are made. Every Sunday morning I eat a waffle topped with fruit and whipped cream (a saturated fat). I do this because I love it! But I can ease my conscience because the waffle is made with nonfat milk and an unsaturated oil, I spray the waffle iron with a nonstick vegetable spray, and I use a very small amount of whipped cream. I choose my poison!

Specific examples of ways to improve the fat composition of your diet are listed in the chart on page 17.

Two other types of food can significantly affect blood lipids. The first is soluble fiber, which is abundant in oat bran, oatmeal, and legumes. Dr. James Anderson of the University of Kentucky has succeeded in dramatically lowering blood cholesterol levels with a diet high in soluble fiber. (See the chapter entitled "Roughing It" for more information on this.) Second, fish oils containing omega 3 fatty acids seem to protect against atherosclerosis. Fatty fish from very cold water regions such as Alaska are the best sources of certain omega 3 fatty acids. Unfortunately the blessing is mixed. Populations consuming large amounts of these fish have fewer heart attacks, but they also have more strokes than Americans. Until we know more about the effects of eating significant amounts of these oils, it is probably unwise to take them as supplements except under a physician's supervision.

Original food	Lower fat	Substitute
Whole milk (4%)	Lowfat milk (1% or 2%)	Nonfat milk
Red meat	• Limit to 3 servings per week • Bake, boil, broil rather than fry • Purchase lean cuts • Remove visible fat	Poultry, fish Legume, pasta, rice entrees
Solid shortening	Decrease amount used	Liquid oil
Hard cheese	Use less	Part skim cheese (check label) Lowfat yellow cheese
Creamed cottage cheese	1% or 2% cottage cheese	Ricotta cheese, part skim Hoop cheese
Egg	Limit to 3 yolks per week In cooking, can use instead of one egg: 1 egg white plus 2 t. oil or 2 egg whites	Egg substitutes Scrambled eggs throw away one third yolks
Butter	Use less	Unsaturated margarine
Mayonnaise	Use less	Low-calorie mayonnaise
Sour cream	Reduced fat sour cream	Plain low or nonfat yogurt

At present, then, I recommend the changes as preventive measures. With a little practice you'll be able to make all of them.

- Limit total fat intake to about 30 percent of total calories (see pages 74-78).
- Limit saturated fat and cholesterol.
- Use twice as much unsaturated as saturated fat.
- Increase soluble fiber.

Our children taught me an important lesson about changing food habits. The issue was milk. All of them had learned to drink nonfat milk after they had passed the age of two (younger children may need the cholesterol in milk). However, I did not like the taste of nonfat milk on cereal, so I continued to buy some lowfat milk even though I rarely ate cereal and milk, and my husband never did (he's allergic to milk). I'd probably still be doing this, but one day the children told me, in simple language that even I could understand, to stop buying lowfat milk. They *liked* nonfat milk! The irony of this interchange struck me, and I realized that here was the kernel of a beautiful truth, which I have never forgotten. It is simply this: Childhood presents a golden opportunity to establish food preferences that promote life and health, and we parents mustn't allow *our* biases to prevent us from doing something wonderful for our children. Simply changing from whole to nonfat milk can drastically cut a child's intake of saturated fat, especially boys, who seem to drink milk by the quart. Almost half of the calories in whole milk are from saturated fat. Almost without exception, even the children's friends who eat at our house happily drink nonfat milk.

Many people who have both high blood pressure and high cholesterol levels can benefit from limiting sodium as well as fat in their diets. If you fall into this category, please refer to the chapter, "Don't get your blood pressure up" (page 29).

If your blood cholesterol level is high and does not respond to dietary change, your physician may prescribe a cholesterol-lowering drug or niacin. These do have side effects, so it is best to try lifestyle changes first.

Chapter 2

Other affairs of the heart

We have discussed the three most important risk factors for coronary heart disease. A number of secondary risk factors have also been identified. These factors are not as powerfully linked with atherosclerosis as are high blood pressure, cigarette smoking, and high blood cholesterol, but they are known to increase a person's chances of developing coronary heart disease. They are:

- Abnormal total cholesterol/high-density cholesterol ratio
- Abnormally high triglyceride levels in the blood
- Obesity
- Physical inactivity
- Stress/personality type
- Diabetes
- Family history of coronary heart disease
- Increasing age
- Male gender

Cholesterol/HDL ratio

We have known for years that measuring the amount of cholesterol in the blood can tell us a lot about the potential development of plaque in the blood vessels. More recently we have learned that all blood cholesterol is not created equal. Let me explain. Because blood has a water base, lipids (cholesterol and all fatty substances) won't dissolve in blood (oil and water don't mix). Therefore, lipids are transported in the blood by combining them with protein. The combined lipid and protein is called a lipoprotein.

While there are many different lipoproteins in the blood, most of the cholesterol is carried by low density lipoprotein (LDL) and high density lipoprotein (HDL). The famous Framingham heart study made the exciting discovery that people with high HDL levels appear to be *protected* against coronary heart disease. We think this is because the HDL carries cholesterol to the liver to be excreted.

As a result of this discovery, total blood cholesterol and HDL cholesterol are now measured, and the ratio between them is calculated. If you have a family history of coronary heart disease or stroke (even if you don't but your total cholesterol is over 200), I strongly recommend that you have your HDL cholesterol as well as your total blood cholesterol measured. Both can be measured from a single blood sample. The ratio between the two is calculated by dividing the total cholesterol number by the HDL cholesterol number. The lower the result the better. In fact, we can be quite specific about the relationship between this number and a person's risk of developing coronary heart disease, provided other risk factors are absent.

Total Cholesterol/HDL Cholesterol Ratio		
Risk of Coronary Heart Disease	**Men**	**Women**
Below average (1/2 average risk)	3.43	3.27
Average	4.97	4.44
Greater than average (twice risk)	9.55	7.05
Greater than average (triple risk)	23.39	11.04

HDL Levels

Below 35 mg% = increased risk
Between 35 and 55 mg% = intermediate risk
Above 55 mg% = low risk

For example, if your total cholesterol is 189 mg% and your HDL cholesterol is 60 mg%, your ratio is 189/60 = 3.15. Comparing this with the chart, you will see that your risk of coronary heart disease is less than half that of the average American. Congratulations! If you don't have any of the other risk factors, skip the rest of this chapter! On the other hand, if your ratio is five or higher, please read on.

Since HDL cholesterol is "good" cholesterol, the next challenge facing scientists was to find out how to move more blood cholesterol out of the LDL type and into the HDL type. Several ways to do this have been uncovered to date. One is exercise. Athletes have high HDL levels. As sedentary people become established in an exercise program, progressively more blood cholesterol is shifted to the HDL side. The total amount of cholesterol in the blood may not change much, but more of it is kept in the protective HDL, which doesn't deposit in the blood vessels.

On the other hand, smoking, obesity, and diabetes tend to lower HDL, while losing weight and quitting smoking increase HDL levels. It has also been noted that HDL levels are raised by drinking alcohol. However, this method of raising HDL is not recommended because of the negative effects of alcohol on the body. Also, drinking alcohol is related to high blood pressure, which is a primary risk factor. Recently it was discovered that monounsaturated oils, like olive and canola oils, lower total blood cholesterol levels without affecting the HDL cholesterol level. This is in contrast to the effect of polyunsaturated oils such as corn, cottonseed, soy, etc., which lower total blood cholesterol but also lower HDL cholesterol levels. The evidence was strong enough to convince me to switch from polyunsaturated to monounsaturated oil in my kitchen.

Up with HDL
Exercise
Reach ideal body weight
Stop smoking
Use olive or canola oil

High triglyceride levels

Now let's look at number two. We've talked a lot about cholesterol, but there is another lipid in the blood that is also routinely measured in order to predict a person's risk of coronary heart disease—triglycerides. These are the true fats. All the fats in foods that we eat are triglycerides, so after eating a fatty meal the blood contains lots of them. This is why a person must fast for several hours before a blood sample is taken to measure triglycerides. You might wonder why there would be any triglycerides in the blood under fasting conditions. Because they are needed to supply the cells with energy. Food is not the only source of triglycerides. The body can also make them from carbohydrate (sugar and starch), protein, or alcohol. In fact, that is what always happens to the extra calories we eat, regardless of where those calories came from originally. Usually these triglycerides are just stored as fat and the person gets fatter! But some families also have a tendency to keep an abnormal level of triglycerides in their bloodstreams.

Under normal fasting conditions there should be 150 milligrams or less of triglyceride in 100 milliliters of blood. There are six distinctly different types of abnormal blood lipid patterns seen in humans. In five of these the triglycerides are much too high—sometimes as high as 6,000 milligrams percent. If your doctor diagnoses you as having one of these disorders it is important to follow his/her recommendations as well as those of a registered dietitian concerning diet. As far as the general population is concerned, it is well to remember that eating a lot of sugar or drinking a lot of alcohol may result in high levels of triglycerides in the blood.

Obesity

I hate the word *obesity*. In my mind it's almost synonymous with anguish, and I know from experience how hard it is to lose weight. But in any discussion of coronary heart disease obesity must be mentioned, because overeating is probably the root cause of many of the lipid abnormalities. The problem is not only eating too much fat, but eating too many calories. Period. Overweight may cause high blood pressure too, which of course is one of the three primary risk factors. The truth is that losing excess weight is critical in the fight against atherosclerosis. For help on how to lose weight and keep it off, see the chapters "Dieting can make you fat" and "Permanent girth control," later in this book.

Physical inactivity

Much has been written about exercise and the prevention of coronary heart disease. It is clear from research findings that sedentary people are more likely than active ones to suffer a heart attack. Exercise of even moderate levels is beneficial. For example, conductors on double-decker buses have significantly fewer heart attacks than do the bus drivers. For exercise to be really helpful it needs to be aerobic—at least twenty minutes three times per week. This kind of exercise will strengthen your heart so that it is more efficient and doesn't have to work as hard.

For instance, if your resting heart rate is seventy-five beats per minute now, it may decrease to sixty or less beats per minute as your fitness level improves. Tiny new blood vessels are also formed which carry oxygen and nutrients to your heart. Even if an artery to the heart becomes blocked, these additional vessels may be sufficient to keep the heart muscle alive. And equally impressive is what exercise can do to blood lipid levels. It can lower total blood cholesterol levels and at the same time increase the HDL (the so-called "good" cholesterol) levels!

Stress and personality type

Stress and personality type go together since a person's stress level is governed by his personality. People can be roughly categorized as either Type A or Type B personalities. People with Type A personalities are ambitious and driven to succeed. They do things quickly and are time conscious. The B personality is more relaxed and tends to take things in stride. Not surprisingly, a disproportionate number of heart attack patients are of the A personality type. But even B personalities suffer the effects of stress in our complex society, and they may also succumb to coronary heart disease. It may seem that there is little we can do to change this risk factor, but actually a number of things can be done.

First we must recognize the *stressors* in our lives that produce *stress* in us. Stressors have different effects on different people. I remember one day when our son Stephen was three years old and we were standing in the checkout line at the supermarket. I was only subconsciously aware that he was singing softly until the checker gave me a pained look that said, "Can't you do something about that child?" I realized immediately that my son's singing bothered her. The stressor (Stephen's singing) produced stress in the checker, whereas it actually had the opposite effect on me. I was Stephen's mother, and if he was happy, I was happy. On the other hand, a floor littered with shoes and socks stresses me, whereas the kids don't mind at all.

It's worth the time to identify the causes of stress in your life, because once you know what they are, you can deal with them. Here are three ways to handle stress. If one doesn't work, try another!

Three ways to handle stress
Avoid
Alleviate
Accept

Avoid. Some stressors can be totally avoided. Maybe the supermarket checker could get a job in a retirement home where there are no little boys! Realistically, though, it is impossible to *completely* avoid all stressors. You can't avoid a demanding boss or a nagging spouse unless you're prepared to walk away and never come back. But often these can be *partially* avoided. For example, the number of stressful *encounters* might be reduced by anticipating and avoiding conflict situations or by learning to communicate better. Anything you can do to reduce the total amount of harmful stress in your life is a step in the right direction.

Alleviate. If stress can't be avoided, there are several ways to alleviate its effects. One is to increase your fitness through regular aerobic exercise. A fit person withstands stress better than an unfit person. Twenty minutes of aerobic exercise three or more times per week is necessary to reap these benefits. See pages 66 to 68 in the chapter "Permanent girth control" for a more complete discussion of what aerobic exercise is and how to monitor it. Exercise is also wonderfully helpful in normalizing the levels of lipids in the blood. Two other tension relievers are to consciously relax and to breathe deeply. Learning to do this takes practice, but both are very effective. And last of all is my favorite way to alleviate stress: laughter. One of the things I love most about my husband is that when everything is going wrong he has the knack of saying something so ludicrous that I dissolve into helpless laughter. A sense of humor may be the best medicine of all!

Accept. Accept is easy to say but hard to do. Life's frustrations tend to yield a crop of negatives like anger and hate. In fact, there is a lot of evidence that hostility is the factor in Type A people which accounts for their high heart attack rate. Finding ways to unload these mental burdens is important. For instance, I love my job, and the very best part about it is getting to know the students well, because we spend so much time together. But once in a while a student does something that makes me mad. It would only make matters worse to blow up at the student, but I can't help feeling angry. Suppressing these feelings escalates stress, so I ventilate my feelings to someone. You can be sure that my husband or maybe one of the kids is going to get a blow-by-blow account that evening of what happened. They may feel bored listening to me, but I feel a lot better.

Dealing with hatred may be even harder than dealing with anger. I wish I could invent a hate eraser, because hate does more to destroy peace and happiness than any other emotion. Hate erodes the spirit, leaving only bitterness. Ironically, the object of the hatred often escapes unharmed. Dealing with such powerful feelings may require professional counseling. The price in time and money can be well worth it.

As a Type A personality myself, what helps me most in living with that which I cannot change is trust in divine power. Life is filled with stress, and it often drains our emotional resources. When this occurs, reaching beyond ourselves for help can make all the difference.

Diabetes
A diabetic person has a significantly greater chance of developing coronary heart disease. But he can reduce that risk by consistently keeping his blood sugar level close to normal.

For overweight type II diabetics (who account for 90 percent of diabetics in the U.S.) the outlook can be even brighter. For many such people, a return to ideal body weight will also cause the high blood sugar levels to normalize.

Regular exercise is important too. Not only does it help in weight control, but it also helps the body to metabolize glucose, which brings the blood sugar level down. If diabetes runs in your family but you have not developed the disease yourself, the most important preventive measure you can take is to achieve and maintain ideal body weight. Your chances of never becoming a diabetic will be vastly improved.

Family history, age, and gender

Coronary heart disease often runs in families. If one or both of your parents had heart disease, your chances of having the same problem are significantly increased. The incidence of heart attack also increases with age, though at a different rate in men than in women. Among American males, heart attacks become increasingly common during the late thirties, and they are rampant after age forty-five. Prior to menopause, heart attacks are seldom seen among American women, but after menopause the incidence of heart attack among women rises till it is equal that of men, and strokes are even more common among women than they are among men.

It is impossible to change or improve your family history, your age, or whether you are male or female. Therefore it is doubly important for those who have these risk factors to lower every other possible risk factor.

The bottom line

When I began studying nutrition in college, the relationship between diet and heart disease was already known. But back in the sixties it was thought that *healthy* Americans didn't need to change their food habits. However, each succeeding year has brought more evidence demonstrating the strong link between lifestyle and atherosclerosis. It is becoming more and more obvious that the American way of life often determines the American way of death. Because of this, in 1988 the American Heart Association published the following nutrition guidelines for all Americans over the age of two years:

1. Total fat intake should be less than 30 percent of calories.
2. Saturated fat intake should be less than 10 percent of calories.
3. Polyunsaturated fat intake should not exceed 10 percent of calories.
4. Cholesterol intake should not exceed 300 mg per day.
5. Carbohydrate intake should constitute 50 percent or more of calories, with an emphasis on complex carbohydrates.
6. Protein intake should provide the remainder of the calories.
7. Sodium intake should not exceed 3 grams per day.
8. Alcohol consumption should not exceed one to two ounces of ethanol per day[1] (two ounces of 100 proof whisky, 8 ounces of wine, or 24 ounces of beer each contain 1 ounce of ethanol), and none at all is far better.
9. Total calories should be sufficient to maintain the individual's recommended body weight.[2]
10. A wide variety of food should be consumed.[3]

I hope this chapter will help you to translate these guidelines into food choices. Whether these goals for America will be achieved remains to be seen. But the fact that American deaths from coronary heart disease are declining indicates that as the critical issues at stake are revealed, more and more Americans *are* choosing the road to high-level wellness.

---

1. I recommend that you not use any alcohol at all.

2. Metropolitan Tables of Height and Weight, Table of Desirable Weights for Men and Women. Metropolitan Life Insurance Company, New York, 1959.

3. "Dietary guidelines for healthy American adults," *Circulation,* March 1988, pp. 721-723.

Desirable Weights for Women Aged 25 and Over

Height With Shoes 2-inch Heels		Small Frame	Medium Frame	Large Frame
Feet	Inches			
4	10	92- 98	96-107	104-119
4	11	94-101	98-110	106-122
5	0	96-104	101-103	109-125
5	1	99-107	104-116	112-128
5	2	102-110	107-119	115-131
5	3	105-113	110-122	118-134
5	4	108-116	113-126	121-138
5	5	111-119	116-130	125-142
5	6	114-123	120-135	129-146
5	7	118-127	124-139	133-150
5	8	122-131	128-143	137-154
5	9	126-135	132-147	141-158
5	10	130-140	136-151	145-163
5	11	134-144	140-155	149-168
6	0	138-148	144-159	153-173

• For nude weight, deduct 2 to 4 lbs. (female).

Desirable Weights for Men Aged 25 and Over

Height With Shoes 1-inch Heels		Small Frame	Medium Frame	Large Frame
Feet	Inches			
5	2	112-120	118-129	126-141
5	3	115-123	121-133	129-144
5	4	118-126	124-136	132-148
5	5	121-129	127-139	135-152
5	6	124-133	130-143	138-156
5	7	128-137	134-147	142-161
5	8	132-141	138-152	147-166
5	9	136-145	142-156	151-170
5	10	140-150	146-160	155-174
6	11	144-154	150-165	159-179
6	0	148-158	154-170	164-184
6	1	152-162	158-175	168-189
6	2	156-167	162-180	173-194
6	3	160-171	167-185	178-199
6	4	164-175	172-190	182-204

• For nude weight, deduct 5 to 7 lbs. (male).

Chapter 3

Don't get your blood pressure up

The heavy door clanged shut, and I stepped into the dim hallway. The unmistakable smell of formaldehyde had been obvious even outside the anatomy building, but here it was overpowering. How I had relished the prospect of studying anatomy! But now that the time had come, my heart was racing, and my mouth felt suddenly dry. I coaxed my feet up the stairs to the laboratory and joined the cluster of students waiting to be assigned a cadaver. Sunshine streamed through the tall windows and fell on the rows of canvas-covered carts where lay the bodies we would come to know so well. Quickly the lab instructor assigned four students to each cadaver, except the last one, where there were only three—Hans, Kathy, and me. Gingerly we pulled back the canvas to reveal the stout, elderly body of a woman. The blood was pounding in my ears as we picked up our scalpels and began to dissect.

The three of us affectionately called her "our body," and as the weeks and months slipped by she opened for us the door of understanding. We stood in awe at the complexity and design of the human body. And as we came to know and understand her muscles, nerves, blood vessels, bones, and organs, I often wondered about *her*. Was her life happy? Did anybody love her? Of course I never knew, but as our skill increased, we learned to see the scars that stress and illness had left behind: the blackened smoker's lungs, the missing gallbladder, the hemorrhage in the brain.

I wish every person with high blood pressure could see the frightful effects this condition can have. It makes the heart beat faster and work harder than it should. It can scar, narrow, and harden the arteries. It can burst a weakened artery in the brain, causing a stroke. It can damage the kidneys. It can cause a heart attack. Maybe seeing these things would make it harder for a person to ignore high blood pressure and hope it will just go away. It never will.

High blood pressure is easy to ignore because there are usually no symptoms associated with it. That's why hypertension is called "the silent killer." Blood pressure must be measured in order to know whether there's a problem. Actually, everyone's blood pressure rises and falls many times during an ordinary day. Mine went up in anatomy lab. That's only natural. The problem comes when the blood pressure *stays* up all the time. Even a garden hose with a weak spot will last a long time if the water pressure inside is kept low. Only when the water is turned on full force does the hose spring a leak. A stroke caused by high blood pressure can be like that. The living brain is delicate, and easily damaged when an artery bursts inside. Brain damage from such a high-pressure hemorrhage has been compared to blasting a fire hose into a room full of whipped cream. If this kind of stroke doesn't kill the person, it often leaves him paralyzed or unable to speak.

How much pressure is too much? A person has hypertension when his blood pressure is above 140/90 millimeters of mercury. The top number (140) is the pressure inside the arteries when the heart is contracting. The bottom number (90) is the pressure when the heart is relaxed. Normal blood pressure is 120/80.

Hypertension won't just go away. It has to be treated. In fact, high blood pressure must be watched and treated for life. But don't despair: it can be controlled, maybe even without medication. The following lifestyle recommendations will help to bring your blood pressure down below 140/90:

> Losing excess weight
> Exercising regularly
> Avoiding or limiting alcohol
> A low-sodium diet
> Eating monounsaturated oils like olive and canola

Antihypertensive drugs are also available, but all drugs have side effects, so it's really worth the effort to work hard on these five lifestyle changes. Let's look at them one by one.

Losing excess weight

The wonderful news is that losing even ten excess pounds can bring blood pressure down significantly. Please read the chapters "Dieting can make you fat" and "Permanent girth control" elsewhere in this book for help. Every excess pound lost is a solid gold investment in your future.

Good luck! I know you can do it!

Exercising regularly

The National Heart, Lung, and Blood Institute recommends the FIT formula for exercise. The "F" stands for *frequency* and means that to be effective you must exercise three to five times per week. The "I" stands for *intensity* and means that the exercise has to be challenging enough to make your heart beat faster (see pages 66 and 67 to learn how to monitor your heart rate). On the other hand, don't overdo it. If you are so breathless that you can't carry on a conversation while exercising, you need to slow down. Brisk walking is great. The "T" stands for *time* and means that each exercise session must last twenty minutes or more.

Limiting or avoiding alcohol

Alcohol tends to increase blood pressure. Any alcoholic drink can have this effect—beer, wine, or hard liquor. If you drink and don't want to quit, at least limit the amount of alcohol you use.

A low-sodium diet

Many people can greatly lower their blood pressure by following a low-sodium diet. Added salt accounts for much of the sodium we eat (40 percent of salt is sodium). One teaspoonful of salt contains 2,000 milligrams of sodium. But sodium is also present naturally in foods. It is used in food processing, and it is found in food additives such as mono-

sodium glutamate. Some medications (certain antacids, for instance) are also high in sodium, so read labels or ask your pharmacist.

Twenty percent of Americans are sodium sensitive. The only way to know whether eating less sodium will help you is to try it. For some people, just a mild sodium reduction helps a lot. For others, extreme restriction is the only answer. Following are some guidelines, starting with a mild sodium restriction and advancing to a strict low sodium diet. (There's practically no danger of going too low; we only *need* 200 milligrams of sodium a day.)

Mild sodium restriction
(3,000-4,000 mg/day)

Don't salt food at the table, use little in cooking.

Avoid very salty foods pickles, olives, bacon, sausage, lunch meats, potato chips, salted crackers, regular canned soups, sauerkraut, ketchup and other sauces (read labels for salt and other sodium sources.)

Moderate sodium restriction
(2,000 mg/day)

Don't salt food in cooking or at the table.

In addition to foods listed above, avoid salted butter, regular salted margarine and mayonnaise, cheese, canned vegetables, salted peanut butter, baked goods made with baking powder, baking soda or salt, instant hot cereals, dry cereals containing 250 mg or more of sodium per serving (check label).

Avoid using more than two cups of milk per day and more than three slices regular bread. Low sodium bread, milk, cheese, etc., may be used as desired.

Strict sodium restriction
(1,000 mg/day)

In addition to the guidelines listed above, avoid carbonated beverages, regular ice cream, more than one egg per day, cottage cheese, milk chocolate, caramel, canned vegetables and juices, frozen vegetables processed with salt, foods containing sodium preservatives or additives.

Commercial salt substitutes (potassium chloride) are OK to use unless you have kidney problems. But always add them *after*, not before cooking, since heat makes them very bitter. There are also several sodium-free herb blends available that you can use both in cooking and at the table. A lot of people like to squeeze fresh lemon over salads, entrees, and vegetables during meals. Lemon adds no sodium, and gives a "bite" similar to that of salt. Remember that tastes change slowly and it usually takes several weeks to adjust to a low sodium diet, so don't despair if you have a hard time at first. Stick with it, and in time you will prefer less salty foods.

Monounsaturated oils
Very recently it has been found that eating monounsaturated oils like olive and canola lowers blood pressure. If you are trying to lose weight you won't be able to use a lot of oil, but even small amounts may be helpful. For several years I bought olive oil (my husband has blood pressure problems), but now that canola is readily available in the U.S. I've switched. The lower cost does *my* Scottish heart good!

Antihypertensive drugs
If your physician prescribes high blood pressure pills, be sure to take them *regularly*. Tell him/her about any unpleasant side effects you may have. There are many different kinds of high blood pressure pills, so you have lots of options.

Something extra for the children

At home I'm doing one other thing as well. We don't know yet whether our children have a tendency toward hypertension. So far so good. But just in case, I try to be sure they get plenty of potassium every day. This means lots of fruit and vegetables, especially fresh ones. There is much evidence that a diet high in potassium protects a person against *developing* high blood pressure.

We also think that a low calcium diet may set the stage for the development of high blood pressure. That gives me another reason to watch the children's calcium intake.

Does it really work?

Stroke is the third leading cause of death in America (after coronary heart disease and cancer). But in recent years the numbers have shifted dramatically. Since 1972, American deaths from stroke have been *cut in half!* Obviously, something wonderful is happening, and we're pretty sure we know what it is. People are smoking less; they are controlling their blood pressure; and they are lowering their blood cholesterol. The National Heart, Lung, and Blood Institute has been conducting a nationwide program of testing and education; physicians are treating high blood pressure more aggressively; dietitians are spreading the good news about nutrition; and the dividends are rolling in! The American people are reaping the rewards in extra golden years.

Chapter 4

Foods that fight cancer

At last nutrition research is bringing into focus the long-suspected relationship between diet and cancer. Since cancer is the second leading cause of death in the United States and one out of every four Americans will develop it at some point during his life, the idea that certain foods might help the body resist cancer brought a glimmer of hope. As evidence accumulated, this possibility strengthened until there emerged a bright certainty that various nutrients do play key roles in defending the body against cancer. It is now clear that diet can enhance cancer resistance.

Four kinds of evidence

Four types of research have helped to build the case for the diet/cancer connection. First, comparing the numbers of cancer cases in different countries aroused the suspicion that there might be a relationship between certain food patterns and the incidence of various cancers. For example, the Japanese living in Japan have a relatively high incidence of cancer of the stomach and eat a lot of smoked fish. On the other hand their diet is low in fat, and their colon and breast cancer rates are low. This is just one example of many apparent relationships seen in different population groups. Such correlations did not *prove* that the food habit *caused* cancer, but they were clues that urged scientists to take a closer look.

More convincing evidence came from noting shifts in types of cancer as a population changed its food habits. As Japanese people migrated to Hawaii and increased their intake of meat and fat and lowered their fiber consumption, their colon and breast cancer rates began to rise. Among Japanese who then settled in the continental United States and adopted the typical American diet, these cancers became even more common. In fact, these people acquired the cancer profile generally seen in the United States. Not only did their incidence of colon and breast cancer rise, but cancer of the stomach declined to the level seen in native Americans.

It was also interesting to find that even subgroups within a given culture showed altered cancer patterns. An example of this is the members of the Seventh-day Adventist Church living in California. The rate of cancer within this group is 40 percent lower than among Californians in general. Members of this church do not smoke, tend to avoid alcohol and caffeine, and many choose a lacto-ovo-vegetarian diet. The lifespan of Adventist men is nine years longer than the California norm. Even more interesting, within this group the vegetarian men live 4.2 years longer than the nonvegetarians.

The second type of evidence comes from animal research. When there is some indication that a certain type of diet may either promote or protect against cancer in humans, this possibility can be tested in animals. Cancer is induced in a group of rats or other animals, and then half the animals are fed a diet rich in the suspected nutrient while the other half get an identical diet except for the nutrient in question. This type of experiment provides more concrete information than do mere human population statistics, because all factors except the one being studied can be held constant. Therefore, any differences between the two groups of animals in the course of the disease and/or length of life can be credited to their diet. Often such animal experiments have confirmed the hunches suggested by human population data.

Yet helpful though animal experiments may be, their results can never be applied directly to humans because of the differences between species. For this reason, a third type of research is most valuable. Actual human cancer cells taken from cancer patients can be kept alive indefinitely in a laboratory setting.

(Normal human cells divide a limited number of times and then die, but cancer cells will continue to divide indefinitely under favorable laboratory conditions.) This makes it possible to investigate how different nutrients influence the rate of growth of cancer cells, because the effect of different nutrients on them can be observed directly in the laboratory.

Of course, the ultimate evidence of the relationship between diet and cancer in humans would be to regulate the diets of healthy people over a period of many years and to compare the number of cases of cancer that develop in different diet groups. This is obviously hard to do. However, there are presently several studies attempting to do this. While it is impossible to control everything that free living people eat like we can with experimental animals, we can increase the intake of a specific nutrient by a study group and compare their cancer rates with those of people eating their usual diets. One of these studies is currently using 30,000 physicians as subjects, and the nutrient being studied is beta carotene. The results should be interesting.

When studies in humans, on animals, and in laboratory cell cultures all point in the same direction, some tentative conclusions can be drawn. It now appears that at least 35 percent of human cancers are diet related. Many specific food patterns have been identified as either helping to promote or to protect against cancer. In order to appreciate their unique roles, some background information about cancer may be helpful.

What is cancer?

Dorland's medical dictionary defines cancer as "a cellular tumor, the natural course of which is fatal." Cancer is usually associated with the formation of secondary tumors. Substances that cause cancer are called carcinogens. There are over a hundred types of cancer, but they can be grouped into five broad categories:

> Carcinomas (those arising from epithelial cells[1])
> Leukemias (blood)
> Lymphomas (lymph system)

Myelomas (bone marrow)
Sarcomas (connective tissue or bone)

It is interesting to note that even though there are many types of cancer, 80 to 90 percent of the human cancer *deaths* in this country are due to carcinomas. All the others put together account for only 10 to 20 percent of cancer deaths. This is probably related to the fact that the epithelial cells which cover and line the body surfaces multiply rapidly, much faster than other types of cells. In fact, cells that seldom multiply, such as nerve cells, rarely become cancerous. This fact will be important in appreciating the role of nutrition in halting the development of cancer.

How does cancer develop?

Cancer apparently begins as a single cell whose genetic code is damaged. As this cell divides, the offspring cells are also abnormal. Eventually, a tumor may develop. Contrary to popular belief, there is usually a prolonged period of time between the first cell damage and actual tumor development—a matter of years or even decades in most cases. But what causes the initial damage to the cell? Carcinogens—chemicals in water or food, compounds in cigarette smoke and other polluted air, certain viruses, and excessive sunlight or radiation from other sources, are just a few that we commonly encounter. Any carcinogen can attack a normal cell and damage its genetic code (DNA).

Stop that carcinogen!

It would be ideal to avoid bringing carcinogens into the body in the first place. We know that stopping smoking is the single best defense against lung cancer because it avoids damage to the lung from tobacco carcinogens. In the same way, avoiding certain cooking methods will prevent the formation of carcinogens on food. When meat is cooked over the heat source and fat drips down onto the coals or stove, carcinogens are formed and carried onto the meat in the rising smoke. Cultures in which people eat a lot of smoked foods or lots of salt-preserved foods have more stomach cancer. Placing aluminum foil or a pan under meat as it is being barbecued is probably a good idea.

Another way to escape carcinogens is to prevent their formation in the first place. This is how vitamin C defends the body from attack by very potent carcinogens called nitrosamines. Nitrosamines are formed in the stomach from nitrates and nitrites, which are present in many foods, water, and even in saliva. Vitamin C can actually stop the formation of nitrosamines.

Of course, vitamin C has to be there in order to act! This bit of knowledge can easily be applied to daily life: Eat some vitamin C at every meal. The meat, milk, and cereal food groups lack this important nutrient, but it is abundant in the fruit and vegetable group. Most fresh fruits and vegetables as well as many cooked ones will do the trick, as long as they have not been cut into tiny pieces and subjected to heat and air, which destroy vitamin C (e.g., potato chips). A piece of cantaloupe at breakfast, a slice of tomato on a sandwich, a baked potato, even strawberry pie, are great ways to accomplish this. Vitamin C may protect us from other carcinogens also, but we *know* that it acts on nitrates and nitrites, to which we are exposed daily.

Inevitably, some carcinogens do get into the gastrointestinal tract, but here again, foods can help. There is good evidence that whole grains contain compounds that are able to detoxify some carcinogens, and a lot of evidence that a high-fiber diet dilutes the concentration of carcinogens in the colon so that they have less chance to act. Incredibly, fiber even helps protect against breast cancer. Vegetarian women have significantly less cancer of the breast, and apparently the credit goes to their higher fiber intake. Breast cancer is related to the level of estrogen circulating in the blood. Estrogens are secreted into the intestinal tract (in the bile), where they can be bound by fiber and then excreted rather than being reabsorbed into the blood. (Be sure to read the chapter on fiber, "Roughing it," later in this book.)

The detoxification center
In spite of everything, some carcinogens do manage to enter the bloodstream, but the body has yet another defense system:

detoxification centers in the liver and other tissues. And again, nutrition is involved. In fact, I think this is the most dramatic food/cancer relationship that has been uncovered. Strong evidence exists to support the conclusion that people who eat generous amounts of cabbage, cauliflower, broccoli, Brussels sprouts, and other vegetables of the cruciferous (cabbage) family have a lower incidence of cancer. Compounds in these foods actually increase the activity of detoxifying enzymes. These enzymes apparently convert carcinogens into harmless compounds, which are then excreted. Unfortunately, as in any detoxification program, not all entering candidates emerge as transformed characters. A few become even more set in their evil ways and leave the detoxification center with enhanced carcinogenic properties. These carcinogens are said to be activated.

Initiation of a normal cell

These activated carcinogens do the dirty work. They attack the genetic material (DNA) within a normal cell and may cause a mutation to occur. All cells resulting from subsequent divisions of this mutated cell will be abnormal. Fortunately, all is not lost just because the DNA has been damaged. Another important nutrient, vitamin A, can play an important protective role. Vitamin A has produced astonishing results in animal experiments, even providing some protection against lung cancer in the presence of cigarette smoke. It has long been known that vitamin A is important in the development of epithelial cells, so it isn't too surprising that it helps the body to resist carcinomas, and possibly sarcomas as well. (Remember that most human cancer deaths are from carcinomas.)

Much human research, including one study on thirty thousand physicians who are taking beta carotene supplements (a precursor of vitamin A), is presently in progress. The verdict is not in yet, but it appears that beta carotene (present in dark green and yellow fruits and vegetables) may be even more effective in cancer prevention than the preformed vitamin A itself (found in animal products like milk, cheese, and egg yolks). At home I keep a bowl of peeled carrots in the refrigerator. They disappear regularly. It's easy to eat some beta carotene daily! Any dark green or yellow fruit or vegetable such as peaches, apricots, broccoli, pumpkin, sweet potato, cantaloupe, etc., is a good source.

Please be aware that an excess of preformed vitamin A can be highly toxic, so vitamin A supplements above the recommended daily allowance are not recommended except under medical supervision. Even too many carotene foods (dark green and yellow fruits and vegetables) can cause a harmless but unattractive yellowing of the skin and whites of the eyes. It's possible to get too much of a good thing, but you would have to eat much more than the recommended one serving per day for this to happen.

Promotion of the damaged cell

Now let's look at the dark side of what happens if the initiated cell is damaged further. This stage is important, because it is probably impossible in the complex world in which we live to completely escape the initiation phase, but promotion may be easier to avoid. Unfortunately, much of the American lifestyle tends to promote the multiplication of damaged (initiated) cells. Some dietary promoters are alcohol, high fat intake, and possibly a high protein intake. A promoter is usually not itself a carcinogen, but it fosters the multiplication of damaged cells over normal ones, creating many more initiated cells, which can again be attacked by carcinogens and be damaged even further.

Tumor development

Cells whose genetic material (DNA) has been damaged in two crucial sites will multiply wildly even without the help of promoters.

Fortunately, all is not lost even at this late stage. In fact, cancer cells probably occur regularly in the bodies of healthy people, but if their immune system is healthy these cells are promptly destroyed. One part of the immune system, the T cell, is specifically delegated to annihilate cancer cells.

Many things help the immune system stay healthy, and

good nutrition is one of the most important. However, obesity causes a drop in the number of killer T cells. Losing extra pounds can bring T cells back up to normal levels.

As far as we know, the immune system is the last of the body's defenses against cancer. If cancer cells are able to elude it, malignant tumors will form. These tumors even send cells into the bloodstream that can start new malignant tumors.

The following recommendations by the American Cancer Society, most of them diet related, should help you to avoid getting cancer.

Eat more cabbage-family vegetables. Important studies show these vegetables (also known as cruciferous) appear to protect you against colorectal, stomach, and respiratory cancers. They include broccoli, cauliflower, Brussels sprouts, all cabbages, and kale.

Add more high-fiber foods. A high-fiber diet may protect you against colon cancer. Fiber occurs in whole grains, fruits, and vegetables, including peaches, strawberries, potatoes, spinach, tomatoes, wheat and bran cereals, rice, popcorn, and whole-wheat bread.

Choose foods with vitamin A. It may help protect you against cancers of the esophagus, larynx, and lung. Fresh foods with beta carotene like carrots, peaches, apricots, squash, and broccoli are the best source, not vitamin pills.

Do the same for vitamin C. This vitamin may help protect you against cancers of the esophagus and stomach. You'll find it naturally in lots of fresh fruits and vegetables like grapefruit, cantaloupe, oranges, strawberries, red and green peppers, broccoli, and tomatoes.

Add weight control. Obesity is linked to cancers of the uterus, gallbladder, breast, and colon. Exercise and lower calorie intake help you avoid gaining a lot of weight. Walking is ideal exercise for most people, and primes you for other sports. However, check with your physician before doing strenuous activity or going on a special diet.

Trim fat from your diet. A high-fat diet increases your risk of breast, colon, and prostate cancer. Fat-loaded calories mean a weight gain for you, especially if you don't exercise.

Cut overall fat intake by eating lean meat, fish, skinned poultry, and low-fat dairy products. Avoid pastry and candies.

Subtract salt-cured, smoked, nitrite-cured foods. Cancers of the esophagus and stomach are common in countries where these foods are eaten in large quantities. Avoid bacon, ham, hot dogs, and salt-cured fish.

Stop cigarette smoking. Smoking is the biggest cancer risk factor of all—the main cause of lung cancer and 30 percent of *all* cancers. Smoking at home means more respiratory and allergic ailments for children. Pregnant women who smoke harm their babies. Chewing tobacco increases the risk of mouth and throat cancers.

Go easy on alcohol. If you drink a lot, your risk of liver cancer increases. Smoking and drinking alcohol greatly increase the risk of cancers of the mouth, throat, larynx, and esophagus. If you do drink alcohol, be moderate.

Respect the sun's rays. Too much sun causes skin cancer and other damage to your skin. Protect yourself with sunscreen (at least #15) and wear long sleeves and a hat, especially during midday hours (11:00 a.m. to 3:00 p.m.). Don't use indoor sunlamps, tanning parlors, or pills. If you see changes in a mole or a sore that does not heal, see your physician.[2]

Postscript

I have outlined in a simple way the process of cancer development as it is initiated by a chemical carcinogen. In doing this, I have run the risk of being misunderstood. The evidence is compelling that the way we eat is intimately and often decisively involved in the success or failure of the body's struggle to ward off cancer—far more than was ever thought possible in simpler times. However, the development of cancer is a complex, multifaceted process, and nutrition is but one of many factors influencing it.

---

1. Skin and mucous membrane that covers the internal and external surfaces of the body.

2. "Taking Control: 10 steps to a healthier life and reduced cancer risk," American Cancer Society, Inc., 1985.

Chapter 5
Roughing it

When I was in second grade a lady came to talk to my class about nutrition. She began by asking, "How many of you eat whole-wheat bread?" The only hand that shot up was mine. Immediately I realized that I had made a mistake. Even at the tender age of seven it was obvious to me that the lady thought I was lying. That afternoon I told my mother what had happened. She was a nutrition-conscious physician and listened sympathetically. Finally she said, "Well, I guess you could have shown her your sandwich!"

Less than thirty years later, how times have changed! One day when our son, Scott, was in the second grade, I packed a white bread sandwich in his lunch. "A nice change from the usual," I thought as I put it in. But at lunchtime a friend stared in astonishment and asked, "Doesn't your mother know that brown bread is better than white bread?"

There are many reasons why whole-wheat bread is superior to white bread, one of which is fiber. Fiber is such a hot topic that scientific journals and popular magazines alike are brimming with articles about it. In fact, fiber has been credited with the ability to save mankind from dozens of maladies ranging from hemorrhoids to cancer. Are any of these claims true, and if so, how much fiber is enough? We don't know all the answers yet, but the mounting evidence is beginning to form an astounding picture of the role of fiber in health.

Even back in the 1800s our foremothers were convinced that what they called "roughage" was good for you, but it was not until 1969 that Dr. Denis Burkett first suggested in the scientific literature that a low-fiber diet might be a cause of colon cancer and a host of other common disorders.

An English missionary-surgeon in Africa, Dr. Burkett noticed that he rarely saw cancer of the colon, hemorrhoids, appendicitis, diverticulitis, phlebitis, gallstones, or even varicose veins among his black African patients, although these conditions were common among his white patients. He came to believe that the high-fiber native diet—rich in vegetables, whole grains, legumes, and fruits—protected them against these diseases. Not sure of the reason, he wondered if fiber might help waste materials pass through the intestines faster, so that carcinogens (cancer-causing substances) weren't in contact with the intestinal wall long enough to do much harm. He also wondered if the larger, more fluid-filled stool produced by a high-fiber diet diluted the concentration of carcinogens.

Since colon cancer kills more Americans than any other cancer except that of the lung, Dr. Burkett's theories set off an intensive search for the truth about fiber and colon cancer. And a number of surprising discoveries have emerged. Fiber does protect against colon cancer, diverticulosis, hemorrhoids, and constipation, and switching to a high-fiber diet actually reverses the proliferation of intestinal polyps, which often turn into cancer.

But the real shockers were unrelated to cancer. To their amazement, scientists found that certain fibers also lower blood cholesterol, sustain blood sugar levels, and facilitate weight loss! Plain, ordinary "roughage" suddenly took on an exciting new importance. Obviously, a major dietary factor had been grossly underrated.

Two kinds of fiber

How could fiber do so many different things? It soon became clear that while there are six kinds of fiber in foods, they fall into two basic categories: water-soluble and insoluble. The insoluble were effective against constipation (and all the problems Dr. Burkett saw) mainly by speeding the mass through the intestinal tract and by retaining its water. On the other hand, soluble fiber forms gels, holds food in the stomach longer, and delays food absorption so that sugar is dispensed more slowly to the bloodstream. The net effect is a lasting feeling of satiety and well-being.

Soluble fiber also binds the cholesterol that the liver secretes into the intestine. Free cholesterol can be easily reabsorbed, but if it is bound to soluble fiber it is excreted instead. The result is less cholesterol in the bloodstream! High-fiber foods also take longer to eat because they need more chewing, and because they are less dense they contain fewer calories. All this helps with weight control.

It became obvious to scientists that both soluble and insoluble fiber are important, and that both are woefully lacking in the typical American diet. In order to gain the benefits of fiber, an adult needs to eat at least twenty grams per day, whereas the average American eats only ten. A glance at the table on page 48 will help you determine how to get enough.

What is fiber, anyway? Fiber is the indigestible part of plants—what's left after digestion is over. Fiber is found in fruits, vegetables, nuts, grains, and cereals, but not in meat, poultry, fish, dairy products, eggs, fats, and sugar. Although fiber makes up a large percentage of stool volume, there are also other kinds of residue left after digestion is completed, as is obvious to anyone who has cared for an infant on a milk diet. But *fiber* is found only in plant foods. Many plants contain both soluble and insoluble fiber; others have mostly one or the other. Good sources of insoluble fiber are whole wheat, most vegetables, and fruits. Oat bran, legumes, and many fruits are rich in soluble fiber.

However, before you rush out to buy oat bran, dried beans, whole grains, and fruits and vegetables, consider this: An abrupt switch from a low- to a high-fiber diet can cause problems. Increase your fiber intake slowly but consistently to give your digestive system a chance to adjust. Otherwise, cramps, bloating, gas, or diarrhea may result. And although you should eventually eat at least twenty grams of fiber every day, more than thirty-five grams per day may hamper mineral absorption. You can get too much of a good thing!

It does your heart good

Soluble fiber's amazing ability to lower blood cholesterol is worth a second thought, especially if your cholesterol level is at or above 300 milligrams percent. People with high cholesterol levels will profit more from soluble fiber than those with cholesterol levels around 200 mg percent, but it's worthwhile for anyone. Oat bran is the soluble fiber that has been studied most, and the results are astounding. Some people have lowered their blood cholesterol 30 percent by eating one cup (measured before cooking) of oat bran daily. One way to get this much is to eat cooked oat bran (half cup dry) as a cereal for breakfast (just cook it like oatmeal) and two oat bran muffins later in the day. You can also add dry oat bran to casseroles, use it instead of flour as breading, and even sprinkle it on top of foods. Remember that most people will need to increase their intake of high-fiber foods *gradually*. Even people with average cholesterol levels can expect a 3 percent decrease by adding one-half cup (measured before cooking) oat*meal* each day. And don't think that oat bran is the only rich source of soluble fiber. Beans, barley, apples, tangerines, and plums are all high in soluble fiber.

An alternative way to bring blood cholesterol levels down with soluble fiber is to use a psyllium laxative (such as Metamucil). Start with one teaspoonful three times a day and increase to one tablespoonful per meal. Psyllium (a grain from western India) contains eight times more fiber than oat bran!

I hope the Fiber in Foods chart will be helpful to you, but I don't really expect you to use it much. Just making small logical changes will suffice. Instead of drinking a lot of juices, eat the whole fruits and vegetables. Or drink juices with pulp rather than those that have been strained. Instead of refined breads and cereals, use whole-grain ones most of the time. As much as possible, eat the skins of fruits and vegetables. Eat at least four servings of breads and cereals and five fruits and vegetables every day. It's worth the effort.

Dietary Fiber in Foods

No Fiber fiber/serving	About 1 gm fiber/serving	2 gm fiber/serving	3 gm fiber/serving	5 gm fiber/serving	High-fiber foods
Eggs Fats and oils Meat, fish, poultry Milk and milk products Sugar and syrups	**Grains** Most cooked cereals (Cream of Wheat, oatmeal) ½ c. Refined cooked cereals (corn flakes, Cheerios, Rice Krispies, etc.) 1 oz. White pasta, ½ c. White bread, 1 slice White flour **Fruits** Fruit juices, ½ c. Grapefruit, ½ c. Watermelon **Vegetables** Asparagus, ½ c. Beets, ½ c. Celery, 1 stalk Cucumber, ½ Green beans, ½ c. Lettuce, 1 c. Radishes, 4 Spinach, ½ c. Summer squash, ½ c.	**Grains** Wheat flakes, ½ c. White rice, ½ c. Whole-wheat pasta, ½ c. **Fruits** Banana, 1 small Cantaloupe, 1 c. Cherries, sweet, ½ c. Dates, 2 Figs, 2 medium Grapes, ¾ c. Mango, ⅔ c. Peach, 1 medium Pineapple, 1 c. Plums, 2 medium Raisins, 3 T. Strawberries, 10 large **Vegetables** Bean sprouts, ½ c. Cabbage, ½ c. Eggplant, ½ c. Green pepper, 1 whole Mushrooms, ½ c. Onions, ⅓ c. Rutabaga, ½ c. Spinach, cooked, ½ c. Tomatoes, 1 small or ½ c. cooked Turnips, ½ c.	**Grains** Cereal with nuts and/or dried fruit, ½ c. Bran cereals, flaked, ½ c. Brown rice, ½ c. Granola, ½ c. Grape-nuts, ⅓ c. Rye, pumpernickel bread, 1 slice Whole-wheat bread, 2 slices **Fruits** Avocado, ½, 3" diameter Blackberries, ⅔ c. **Vegetables** Beans, lima, ½ c. Broccoli, ½ c. Brussel sprouts, ⅓ c. Cabbage, ½ c. Carrots, ⅓ c. Cauliflower, ½ c. Kale, ⅓ c. Potato, ½ medium or ½ c. Sweet potato, 1 small or ½ c.	**Grains** Cracklin' Oat Bran cereal, ⅔ c. Barley, dry, ¼ c. **Fruits** Apple with skin, 2" diameter Blueberries, ⅔ c. Coconut, shredded, ¾ c. Orange, 1 large with membrane Pear with skin, 2-½" diameter Raspberries, ¾ c. **Vegetables** Beans, pinto, kidney, ½ c. Corn, 4" ear or ½ c. Lentils, cooked, ⅔ c. Peas, green, ½ c. **Nuts** Almonds, ⅓ c. Brazil nuts, ½ c. Peanuts, ½ c. Pistachio nuts, ½ c. Walnuts, ¾ c.	All-Bran cereal ½ c. = 8 gm fiber Bran, unprocessed, 3 T. = 4 gm fiber 40% Bran Flakes cereal, ½ c. = 4 gm fiber 100% Bran cereal (Nabisco) ½ c. = 10 gm fiber Fiber One cereal, ½ c. = 13 gm fiber

To find grams of fat and calories per serving, read labels.

gm fat/serving x 9

Chapter 6

The great bone robbery

A couple walked by as I stood waiting at Los Angeles International Airport, and I overheard the woman say, "Well, you know we shrink when we get older, and she never was that tall."

Was she right? Do people lose height as they age? Are the expressions "little old ladies" and "little old men" rooted in fact?

Here in the United States the answer is too often Yes, especially for women. And the underlying problem is usually osteoporosis. Simply stated, this means that the bones are slowly robbed of calcium until they can no longer tolerate ordinary stress. A hug can break a rib. A fall can fracture a hip. Spinal vertebrae may collapse, causing a "dowager's hump." Even the jawbone can become too thin to hold teeth or support dentures. And saddest of all, young Americans are unknowingly setting themselves up to lose big in the skeleton sweepstakes.

Bare bones facts

Everybody knows that babies and young children need lots of calcium, because their teeth and bones are obviously forming. But the truth is that bones continue to become thicker, heavier, and stronger until age twenty-five for vertebrae and forty for arms and legs. Between 10 and 15 percent of bone mass is added between ages twelve and forty. But sometime in the fourth decade of life, the process reverses and the bones start to thin. This happens regardless of race, sex, or lifestyle. It's inevitable. In time the bones may become so brittle that

49

they fracture easily. That's osteoporosis. This condition is so common in the United States that billions of dollars are spent annually treating the resulting fractures. My own father was an orthopedic surgeon, and he essentially put my two sisters and me through college by setting broken hips! And 20 percent of hip fracture victims die within the following year.

Women are more vulnerable to osteoporosis because they build less bone while they're growing up and lose it faster after the menopause. But men get osteoporosis too, and the first clue in either sex is a fracture. You can't feel the bones weakening. There are ways to measure bone density, but they're not easy or cheap. In fact, usually only university hospitals have the necessary equipment. Only in recent years has it been possible to partially rebuild the thinned bone, and at best the process is slow, very expensive, and not always successful.

There is hope

Even though bone loss is unavoidable, the situation is anything but hopeless. Prevention is the key, and the most important factor by far is building a dense, strong skeleton early in life. In fact, for some unknown reason, not more than 45 percent of the calcium is withdrawn from the bones no matter how long a person lives. You can't lose all of your bones! Therefore a person with very dense bones to start with can stay out of the fracture range for life because he can afford to lose 40 percent of the calcium in his bones and still have bones solid enough to withstand normal stress. Of course, if he plays tackle football at age seventy-five, something might give, but we're talking about the strains of ordinary life.

Two things are essential to achieve maximum bone density while the bones are forming: calcium and exercise. Looking at the eating and exercising patterns of young Americans sheds a lot of light on why more women than men have osteoporosis. For one thing, girls eat a lot less calcium than boys. In fact, most males in the United States consume the recommended daily allowance (RDA) for calcium until about age sixty. Girls do well, too, until they become teenagers, but then it's downhill all the way. During the critical years of eighteen to twenty-four the average American girl is actually taking in only a little more than *half* the RDA for calcium. Exercise habits vary too. Males tend to exercise more. American women seem to make one of two mistakes—too little exercise or too much. Weight-bearing exercise like walking or jogging seems to produce a charge like static electricity inside the bones, which stimulates bone growth. Inactivity has the opposite effect. Astronauts lose calcium from their bones while in space due to the weightless conditions. So we know that exercise is important in building strong bones, but we're not sure exactly how much is needed. We do know that women who train so hard that they stop menstruating *lose* bone mass because estrogen protects the bones. So either extreme is damaging. But frequent weight-bearing exercise is probably more important to building a sturdy skeleton than any factor other than eating plenty of calcium.

Let's assume that childhood diet and exercise weren't so great early on. The person has marginal bone density when he reaches age thirty-five, and bone loss begins. Can anything be done to slow the process? Yes! Calcium and exercise are still crucial. For a lot of reasons. With aging, the body doesn't absorb calcium as well. Older people may also avoid sunlight, so they may be deficient in vitamin D, which facilitates calcium absorption. Caffeine, alcohol, smoking, and a high-protein diet promote calcium excretion, so you can see that the American lifestyle is a liability. Therefore a generous calcium intake is critical—at least the recommended 800 mg per day. Exercise is still important too. In fact, loading exercise (like walking, which stresses the bones) can actually increase bone density even in older people. Swimming doesn't seem to work since it isn't weight bearing. Both calcium and exercise are important in both sexes.

For post-menopausal women, one other thing can help dramatically: estrogen replacement, especially during the first five to ten years following menopause, when bone loss is fastest. Since high-dose estrogen therapy has been linked to cancer of the uterus, low doses are used now. Also, if calcium intake is high (1,500 mg per day), some evidence suggests that really small amounts of estrogen will still protect the bones. In any event, it's important to be closely followed by a competent physician when on estrogen therapy.

The bottom line

I've tried to build a strong case for a generous calcium intake throughout life because the evidence points convincingly in that direction. I know that there are populations on low-calcium intakes who have less osteoporosis than Americans do, but the fact that they do more manual labor, have more exposure to sunlight, and especially, that they eat a lower protein diet probably accounts for the difference.

The U.S. calcium RDA for adults is set at 800 mg per day, but many nutritionists think that's too low. Post-menopausal women should probably aim for 1,200 to 1,500 mg per day. A cup of milk or yogurt, or an ounce and a half of cheese, or 1 ½ cups of ice cream or cottage cheese have about 300 mg of calcium. Nondairy foods are much lower. Tofu (2 oz.), canned salmon with bones (3 oz.), broccoli, turnip, or kale (half cup) all have about 100 mg of calcium. If you drink two cups of milk a day you probably reach the RDA of 800 mg even if you eat no other dairy products, because almost all foods have a little calcium in them. People who don't use dairy products may need a calcium supplement. Calcium carbonate (such as Tums antacid) is 40 percent calcium, dibasic calcium phosphate is 29 percent, calcium lactate is 13 percent, and calcium gluconate is 9 percent. Calcium carbonate causes constipation in some people, so calcium lactate or gluconate may be preferred. Also, the supplement should be taken in divided doses to be well absorbed. And drink lots of water if you're taking a supplement, especially if you're prone to kidney stones. Getting the calcium from food is really better!

But the important thing is to get it. Because the great bone robbery is for real.

Chapter 7

Alcohol and pregnancy

"A jug of wine, a loaf of bread—and thou." When Omar Khayyam wrote these words, he tried to convey a sense of the deep delight that a man and woman can find in each other. As contemporary filmmakers and writers try to do likewise, they often use similar scenes. Whether the setting is under a tree in a grassy meadow, or a soft carpet by an open fire, wine, champagne, or other alcoholic beverages are often there. When Khayyam said "thou" he referred to a beautiful woman. But I would like to change the meaning to refer to an unseen and perhaps unknown individual who may be present, and on whom alcohol can have catastrophic consequences: an unborn child.

Alcohol has been consumed throughout recorded history. Yet not until 1973 did the medical profession awaken to the fact that drinking alcohol during pregnancy can result in irreversible birth defects. Dr. David W. Smith, a Seattle pediatrician, noticed that babies born to alcoholic women often had certain characteristic malformations, and that as they grew into childhood they were frequently mentally retarded. He called this group of symptoms "fetal alcohol syndrome."

Long ago in the Hebrew Scriptures the story was told of an angel appearing to the future mother of Samson. The angel said, "Thou shalt conceive, and bear a son; and now drink no wine nor strong drink" (Judges 13:7). Both Aristotle and Plutarch noted that alcoholics begat children resembling themselves. Even the British novelist Charles Dickens noted that the children born to women who drank heavily were often

53

mentally retarded. Nevertheless, Dr. Smith was the first physician to describe a unique group of defects seen in eleven children, and to suggest that they were the result of their mothers' alcohol intake during pregnancy.

Effect of alcohol during pregnancy

Almost two decades have passed since fetal alcohol syndrome was first described in the scientific literature, and many questions about it remain unanswered, but several of its aspects have become clear. Among these are the following:

- The defects are permanent.
- Alcohol itself (apart from cigarette smoking, caffeine, drugs, etc.) causes the abnormalities.
- The amount of alcohol necessary to produce the condition varies according to the metabolism of the pregnant woman and that of her unborn child. Three sets of nonidentical twins have been reported in which one was normal and the other had all the physical defects.
- The level of alcohol in the mother's blood is the critical factor. High blood alcohol levels in the father at conception apparently do not cause fetal alcohol syndrome.
- The severity of defects varies among victims. The effect on the child is related to both the peak levels of alcohol in the mother's blood and the amount of time during the pregnancy that she drank.
- Binge drinking can cause fetal alcohol syndrome. Relatively moderate blood levels of alcohol can result in a child who may have only a few of the characteristics of fetal alcohol syndrome. These children are described as suffering from fetal alcohol effects.

Characteristics of fetal alcohol syndrome

What were the characteristics that Dr. Smith saw in his eleven patients? The complete syndrome encompasses a constellation of symptoms, three of which are abnormalities of the head and face, retarded growth before and after birth, and mental retardation.

The most obvious characteristics are the facial abnormalities. The head is small with closely set eyes. The inner corners of the eyes are covered by a fold of skin like that present in Orientals. The bridge of the nose is virtually nonexistent, and the nose itself is short and upturned. The two ridges that usually extend from the nose to the upper lip are absent or poorly developed, and the upper lip is thin.

Intelligence is often directly proportional to the severity of the facial defects. The number of physical abnormalities and the degree of mental impairment usually go hand in hand. Other less common characteristics that are frequently seen include crossed or "wandering" eyes, poorly formed, low-set ears, small teeth with thin enamel, heart defects, abnormal creases in the palms of the hands, and various bone and joint defects.

A child with the full-blown fetal alcohol syndrome usually has all the facial characteristics and may also have several of the less common defects. Mental retardation ranges from mild to severe, with I.Q.s as low as 50 compared to the average normal I.Q. of 100. Less damaged children may show none of the physical abnormalities but may have learning problems, especially concentration difficulties, in school.

Ten years after Dr. Smith diagnosed his first eleven cases of fetal alcohol syndrome, he followed up on eight of them. Four of these had borderline intelligence and required remedial teaching, and four were severely retarded and needed constant supervision.

Safe levels of alcohol intake during pregnancy

So how much alcohol can a woman safely drink during pregnancy? The answer isn't clear, but the following conclusions seem clear from animal experiments.

- The equivalent of one drink (1-1/2 oz. hard liquor, 12 oz. beer, 4-5 oz. wine or 3 oz. sherry) per day has no demonstrable effect on the fetus.
- Two drinks per day result in an increased number of offspring who appear normal physically but have learning difficulties as adults.

- Three drinks per day increase the number of fetal deaths.
- Four drinks per day increase the likelihood of low birth weight and size, which persist into later life.
- Five drinks result in many offspring who have the characteristic malformations of the fetal alcohol syndrome.

Animal experiments like these are helpful, but it is dangerous to make direct application to humans. We really do not know what amount of alcohol, if any, is safe for a woman to drink during pregnancy. The harmful effects on the baby depend on the metabolism of both the mother and the child. Animal experiments indicate that high blood alcohol levels immediately prior to conception *may* also be detrimental. The safest course is to abstain from drinking any alcohol before, and especially during, pregnancy. Women who are unable to stop drinking on their own should seek help before becoming pregnant. A number of studies show that even if a woman has been drinking during pregnancy, her child will benefit if she stops drinking even as late as the third trimester.

It doesn't have to happen

We don't know just how common fetal alcohol syndrome is. Physicians are diagnosing it more frequently as they become more familiar with its characteristics, but sometimes these aren't easy to detect in a newborn or even in an older child. The syndrome is most easily recognized in the preschool child. The tragedy is that it ever occurs. No child need suffer these lifelong handicaps. *The condition is 100 percent preventable.*

So in concluding this chapter I would like to give voice to those who cannot speak for themselves—the unborn and those not yet conceived. For them I would like to say, "If you give me life, let it begin without limitations. Allow me the capacity to comprehend the recorded wisdom of ages past; to appreciate the beauty in nature, art, and music; to reason logically; to excel in sports; to create something unique and beautiful; to perceive the nuances in human interaction so that I may build lasting, loving relationships.

"Please, give me that chance."

Chapter 8

Dieting can make you fat

I first went on a reducing diet when I was twelve. I weighed in at 118 pounds, and I wanted to weigh 115. That was over thirty years, three term pregnancies, and countless reducing diets ago. This morning I weighed 115. There were months and even years in between when finding time to step on a scale was hard, but one day I did, and I was jolted into facing reality. *One hundred forty-five pounds!* How could this have happened to me, a person educated in clinical nutrition, no less? The answer was simple. The same way it happens to most people. Slowly. Almost imperceptibly. As I looked at that scale, I knew the time had come to apply the knowledge in my head to my own life.

The weight came off the same way it went on. Slowly.

But was it worth the effort? Did an advanced education in nutrition alter my method of girth control? Yes, on both counts. In fact my ideas about weight management have changed a lot as a result of new discoveries about energy balance. My face gets red when I think of some of the people I counseled on low-calorie diets twenty-five years ago. Back then I was confident that as long as I taught them how to keep their calorie intake below maintenance level they would lose weight. After all, a person's weight was simply a reflection of the balance between the energy taken in (energy in) and the energy expended (energy out), or so I thought.

So I concentrated on teaching people how to keep their calorie intake (energy in) down. I seldom mentioned changing the energy expended. I assumed that would remain the same. When some clients came back later and told me they had followed the diet and hadn't lost much weight, I thought they were cheating and were really eating more calories than allowed. I wish I could go back and apologize. It was almost like giving a beginner one ski and expecting him to make it down the hill. I still believe that weight reflects the balance between "energy in" and "energy out," only now I know that "energy out" is far more complex than we once thought. A successful weight control program should take both sides of the equation into consideration. If you don't, you may join the thousands of Americans who diet and lose weight but regain it almost as fast. The awful truth is that *dieting can make you fat*. If you lose and regain repeatedly, it can even leave you fatter than before you began losing weight in the first place. But don't despair. We've also learned how to achieve permanent weight control.

But first there are some basics every weight loss hopeful needs to know.

Where does "energy in" come from?

"Energy in" simply means the number of calories we eat. Humans can get energy only from food. Calories are a way to measure energy, and they come from only four sources: carbohydrates (starches and sugars), protein, fat, and alcohol. The number of calories from these sources varies a lot. In one gram of each (454 grams = 1 lb.) there are:

Carbohydrate (starches and sugars)	4 calories
Fat	9 calories
Protein	4 calories
Alcohol	7 calories

Many foods are a combination of energy sources. For example, meat contains both protein and fat. Cake contains carbohydrates, fat, and a little protein. The calories in a given food reflect the relative amounts of the four energy sources in it. So the number of calories taken in can be decreased by eating *less* food *or* by eating the same *quantity* of food but less fat and alcohol.

What is "energy out"?

Let's go back to our original equation. We've established that "energy in" is composed entirely of calories from food eaten. But what about "energy out"? "Energy out" can be divided into three parts:

> Basal metabolic rate (BMR),
> Thermic effect of food (TEF),
> Muscle energy expenditure (MEE).

Basal metabolic rate is the energy the body uses just to maintain life: breathing, beating of the heart, maintaining body temperature. Thermic effect of food is the energy used to digest and utilize food. Muscle energy expenditure is the energy used in physical exercise. An average person whose weight is stable uses about 60 percent of his energy for basal metabolic rate, 10 percent for thermic effect of food, and 30 percent for muscle energy expenditure. Notice that the basal metabolic rate accounts for more than half of the total calories used. You'll see how important this is later.

The bad news about "energy out"

As far as weight control is concerned, there is good news and bad news from energy research. The bad news is that when calories eaten (energy in) are decreased, the body responds by lowering energy out. It uses fewer calories for basal metabolic rate and thermic effect of food. When you give it less energy, the body responds by using less energy for its basic operations. It becomes more energy efficient. This is a protective mechanism of life-saving importance under starvation circumstances, but it can be devastating to the dieter, because the very act of decreasing "energy in" can reduce "energy out," so that the net energy deficit is small and little weight is lost.

This phenomenon explains why some of my clients really *were* following the low-calorie diet I prescribed and still failed to lose much weight.

Fortunately, this starvation-induced reduction of "energy in" is limited, so when calories are sharply reduced, weight loss will occur. But there's a price to be paid. Drastically reducing the calories in results in a big drop in basal metabolic rate. There is even evidence that people who repeatedly go on very low calorie diets may permanently lower their basal metabolic rate. This means that returning to a moderate calorie intake will result in a weight *gain*. I know women who can no longer eat 1,200 calories a day without gaining weight because of this kind of yo-yo dieting. This is just one reason why I do not usually recommend very low calorie diets (below 1,000 calories per day for most women or 1,200 calories per day for most men). Another reason relates to the ultimate body composition following semistarvation diets. But more about that later.

For these reasons, the very low calorie diets (400 to 800 calories per day) should be used only when fifty or more pounds must be lost, and then only under the supervision of a physician. In those cases obesity may be more harmful than the semistarvation diet. Deaths resulting from prolonged, extreme calorie restriction (usually about 400 calories per day) have almost all been due to heart failure. For this reason, electrocardiograms should be done regularly on anyone following a very low calorie diet for more than a short time. Also, on any diet lower than 1,200 calories per day it is a good idea to take a multivitamin supplement containing *no more than 100 percent of the U.S. recommended daily allowances*. Premenopausal women should choose a supplement that also contains iron.

The good news about "energy out"

But let's get back to the problem of the body's cutting back on the calories used when few calories are consumed. That brings us to the good news from energy research. Simply put, it is this: exercise can *increase* "energy out" in two ways. First, it burns extra calories during the exercise itself, and second, it increases the basal metabolic rate and thermic effect of food. The really great news is that following aerobic exercise there is a *prolonged* increase in energy expenditure by the body. Even after the exercise ends, the body's metabolic rate remains high, so excess calories continue to be burned. How long this effect lasts appears to be related to the amount of lean body mass in the person doing the exercise. The more muscle, the more calories used. So things get better and better as your fitness improves.

Making "energy out" work for you

This knowledge has changed my own weight control program. Now, when I need to lose weight, I curtail calories moderately, but I also exercise once or twice a day. At first, making myself exercise wasn't easy. I spent my academic career avoiding physical education, so exercise held all the appeal of having a root canal! Ten years ago I couldn't run a mile, and I really didn't want to. Now I jog more than that every morning. I wouldn't have believed that I would ever say this, but I really enjoy it. In fact I feel cheated when work or family duties prevent me from going.

Each season has its own delights. The bright autumn leaves in the golden sunlight. Snowy mountains in winter. Springtime air heavy with the sweetness of orange blossoms. Deep pools of shade cast by the giant trees in summer. I come home filled with peace. It's a marvelous, "God's in His heaven, all's well with the world" sort of feeling. The crowded day ahead seems manageable. Of course, I'm lucky to live in a small California town, but I've also jogged in big cities, and there's beauty there too.

Another surprising side effect of exercise is that instead of sapping energy, it gives me more! I feel more alive. This natural "high" comes from the endorphins (morphinelike compounds) produced by the body during exercise, as well as from the increased oxygen supply to body tissues. The effect lasts for many hours after the exercise has ended.

Don't get me wrong. Exercise isn't a shortcut to quick weight loss. In fact, as body fat is lost and lean body mass is increased, there may be little change in actual weight for a while. Lean body mass (75 percent water) weighs more than fat (19 percent water). But you will begin to look better at the same weight, and even better as jiggly fat is slowly replaced by smooth, firm muscle. I'll never forget buying a size six dress again for the first time in years!

The benefit of exercising while dieting was well illustrated by a group of overweight people who went on a 1,000-calorie-a-day diet. Half of them also walked for thirty minutes each day. The other half didn't do any exercise beyond their normal daily activities. At the end of two months the "diet only" group had lost twenty pounds, and the "diet-walking" group had lost twenty-three pounds. Not a very impressive difference over a two-month period. However, the difference in body *composition* between the two groups was dramatic. Eight of the twenty pounds the "diet only" group had lost were muscle and twelve were fat. The "diet-walking" group had *gained* two pounds of muscle and lost twenty-five of fat. They lost over *twice* as much fat as the "diet only" group!

Why do we care about body composition? Appearance, for one thing. Muscle is firm and smooth and gives the body curves. Fat is lumpy and shapeless. But even more important for weight control, the future is much brighter for a person with more lean body mass. Fat burns calories slower than the same amount of muscle, so the "diet only" group will gain their weight back much more easily, on fewer calories, than the "diet-walking" group.

Slow weight loss for the long haul

This brings us to another important point. Slow weight loss is much more likely to be permanent. The rapid initial loss on a semistarvation diet (400 to 800 calories per day) is not all fat. It is part fat, part lean body mass, and largely water. About 50 percent of a woman's weight and 60 percent of a man's is water. Six or more pounds can be quickly shed within a few days on a very low calorie diet without significantly reducing body fat. Quick weight loss is often followed by regaining most or all of the pounds lost. Repeating the cycle makes matters worse. One group of eighty obese people lost an average of forty-eight pounds in 232 days, averaging .26 pounds per day on a very low calorie liquid diet. Later, after regaining the lost weight, they tried the same program again since it had proved so successful before. This time they averaged a loss of twenty-four pounds in 187 days—an average of .16 pounds per day, which was much less than before. Apparently the rapid lose/gain/lose cycle made it progressively harder to lose weight each time and easier to regain it. In fact, it took almost twice as long to lose the same amount of weight the second time around. Another very important point is that both muscle and fat are lost on a crash diet, but the weight quickly regained is mostly fat. Since a pound of fat is more bulky than a pound of muscle, clothing sizes climb after a quick loss/regain cycle, even if the initial and final *body weights* are the same.

Stick with me

Now you know that I think quick weight loss is a little like shooting yourself in the foot. But I know that many of you will choose this tempting option rather than slow weight loss, which I will describe in the next chapter. Please read it anyway, because no matter how you *lose* weight, *keeping* it off will depend on changing your "fat habits" to "skinny habits." Trust me on this one. It's true. I'll tell you how to do it in the next chapter.

Chapter 9

Permanent girth control

It's terribly discouraging to look at weight control program statistics. The failure rate often approaches 95 percent! Many people successfully *lose* weight, but few are able to *keep* it off. Many reasons exist for this sad state of affairs, some related to inheritance and some to repeated "crash" dieting. But one factor outshines all others: "fat habits" were never changed. Oh, the person changed his eating habits for a while—a few days or weeks perhaps, or even months. But when the goal had been reached, he or she went back to the old "fat" habits, and the weight came back on.

This doesn't have to happen. It is possible for you to lose weight and keep it off through realistic changes in eating and exercise patterns that you will come to value so much that you won't want to go back to the old ways. My experience with exercise is an illustration of this phenomenon. Whereas I once hated jogging, I now value it so much that I never want to be inactive again. I have completely reversed my attitude about exercise.

How did this radical change in my thinking come about? The answer is clear and simple. If you can follow a recipe, you can do it.

We now know that a person won't value a behavior enough to incorporate it permanently into his life until he goes through seven stages. The desired *goal* is irrelevant. Whether you want to learn to play the violin, to become fluent in German, or to achieve permanent weight control, the steps are the same.

Seven essential steps

First, you must become aware of a need for change. Since you are reading this chapter, you have probably already taken this step. You know that you need to lose weight.

Second, you must acquire knowledge about how to make the change. The latter part of this chapter will describe the actions you must take to lose weight.

Third, you must repeat these actions many times. You must practice the techniques. Unfortunately, here is where most people stop. At first the new behaviors are strange, and it's easy to fall back into old habits. Getting beyond this step greatly increases your chances for success.

Fourth, as a result of practice, you will become capable. The new behavior doesn't seem difficult any longer. Practice has made it come naturally.

Fifth, with capability you will gain a positive attitude about the new behaviors. You will enjoy doing them!

Sixth, you will now be motivated to continue your new life-style indefinitely. Are you surprised to find motivation at this point? Usually we think of motivation coming *before* a person starts to change, and indeed, in the beginning there is a desire to reach a certain goal. But the motivation to *continue* the new behaviors won't come until the first five steps have been taken.

Finally you will reach the seventh step—valuing the new behavior. You will cherish this new lifestyle, and you won't want to go back to your former way of life. These new behaviors will be truly important to you. Those who reach this seventh step achieve a permanent lifestyle change. Going through all seven steps takes time, which is another reason why permanent weight loss is usually slow. Now let's apply this seven-step process to the problem of weight reduction.

Awareness

Becoming aware of the advantages of achieving ideal body weight is easy in our culture. Health reasons abound. Coronary heart disease, certain cancers, high blood pressure, adult-onset diabetes, stroke, gout, gallstones, varicose veins, and many other conditions are strongly correlated with overweight.

I frequently lecture on obesity-related diseases, and I often see such patients in the hospital, but I watch my own weight for more immediate rewards: buying clothes in sizes that look good; keeping up with our three teenagers; enjoying my husband's approval. These are a few of the reasons that keep me exercising and watching my diet.

Whatever *your* goal may be, having it clearly in mind is important. Rather than setting a weight goal, it's better to aim for a certain size of clothes. As I mentioned before, a loss of body fat and a simultaneous increase in lean body mass won't show up on the scale for a while, but the results will be visible in the clothes you wear!

Knowledge

The knowledge necessary for permanent weight control can be divided into two categories: food facts and exercise facts. Let's discuss food first.

By far the most important technique in limiting calories is to reduce fat intake. Fat has nine calories per gram—more than twice as many as protein and carbohydrate, both of which have four calories per gram. Eating less fat also reduces your risk of cancer and heart disease. Therefore it is essential to recognize the fat in foods. Some fats are obvious: butter, margarine, cream, mayonnaise, salad dressing, sour cream, cream cheese, oils, shortening, and lard. Other fats are less obvious: olives, nuts, bacon, and avocado, to name a few. You don't have to *eliminate* these foods, but they must be *limited*. Hidden fats are the greatest challenge. Refer to the Fats of Life chart to get a feel for the fat content of various foods. Alcohol is also high in calories—seven calories per gram—and sugar is a concentrated calorie source. But more on this later.

Now for some exercise facts. Duration and intensity of exercise are both important in order to build muscle and boost the metabolic rate. The goal is to exercise once or twice daily for fifteen to twenty minutes at aerobic intensity. "Aerobic" means that the oxygen used by the body tissues has been significantly increased. You can know when you are exercising at aerobic levels by your heart rate. Subtract your age from 220, and then take 70 to 80 percent of that number. A forty-five-year-old would have a target exercise heart rate of 122 to 140. That's the number of times per minute his heart should beat during aerobic exercise.[1] The following diagram illustrates these figures:

220	220
-45 age in years	-45 age in years
175	175
x .70 (70%)	x .80 (80%)
122	140

To monitor your heart rate you will need a stopwatch or a watch with a second hand. Immediately after you stop exercising, take your pulse at your wrist for ten seconds. Multiply this by six to get your heart rate per minute. Count for only the first ten seconds, because your heart begins to slow down immediately after you stop exercising, and you want to estimate your heart rate during exercise. I have just described the most accurate way to know whether your exercise is intense enough to really do some good.

Actually, I don't use this method myself. One reason is that I don't have a second hand on my watch, and another is that there is an easier way to do it that is pretty good. A simple rule of thumb is to exercise at a level that makes you break out in a light sweat and moderately speed up your breathing— but not so much that you are unable to talk.

Respiration and perspiration are quite reliable guides.

Getting started

Do you feel tired just reading the previous few paragraphs? Are you thinking that maybe you like yourself the way you are, and that the kind of exercise I have described is worse than wearing a size twenty? Take heart. It isn't so bad. Although I exercise for twenty-minute stints now, I certainly didn't start that way. Ten minutes of walking once a day is a beginning. For many overweight people, walking is aerobic. Gradually increase the intensity of exercise five minutes per session after a week. If you are over thirty-five and have been sedentary, have a physical examination before starting an exercise program.

The important thing is to get started.

Two fifteen-minute sessions morning and evening are better than one session twice as long, because you boost your metabolic rate after *each* exercise period! Besides, it's easier to carve fifteen or twenty minutes out of a busy schedule. When I absolutely can't leave the house or stop to exercise, I jog in place. Our children have watched me jogging in place while doing so many things (cooking breakfast, sewing on buttons) that Stephen felt compelled to warn me against trying it while painting! (He meant walls, not pictures. The house we live in is a hundred years old, and the kids will forever remember me with a paintbrush in my hand.) The point is that we all have little pockets of time that can be captured.

Equally important is finding an activity that you enjoy. Otherwise you probably won't stick with it. A warm-up (stretching) at the beginning and a cool-down (slow movement) period at the end of each exercise session will help to prevent undue stress on your body. If you are very overweight, you will need to avoid weight-bearing impact exercise like jogging until you've lost some weight. Appropriate nonweight-bearing exercises include walking, swimming, and cycling. Whatever exercise you choose, be sure to begin slowly, and gradually increase the duration and intensity until you are exercising for at least twenty minutes per session at an aerobic level. To make a real difference, exercise at least once and preferably twice per day while losing weight.

Practice

When I say practice I mean the act of performing a behavior repeatedly. Applied to weight control this means behaviors having to do with eating and exercising. We have listed the foods to limit (fats, sugar, and alcohol) and how to exercise. So now it's just a matter of going out and doing it, right? If only it were that easy! Unfortunately, habits of many years do not relinquish their stranglehold without a fight. It takes time. Let me share some techniques that work. Every "fat habit" needs to be replaced with a "skinny habit." Here's a list of some "skinny habits" to be acquired.

Skinny habits

1. Eat three meals a day and don't snack in between.
2. Sit down at a table to eat. Don't eat standing up.
3. Limit fats.
4. Limit sugar.
5. Limit or eliminate alcohol.
6. Eat slowly, and don't put more food on your fork until you have swallowed the food in your mouth.
7. Don't take a second helping until fifteen minutes after the first. Even better, don't eat seconds.
8. Don't read or watch TV while eating. (Enjoy the food!)
9. Eat in a pleasant place and make the food look pretty on the plate.
10. Exercise at least twenty minutes daily at an aerobic level.
11. Stand nude in front of a full-length mirror every morning.

Now, let's say you're really ambitious and decide to incorporate the first two behaviors for a whole week. That's what I decided to do, because I didn't snack very much anyway, and I thought that sitting down to eat should be easy. Was I ever wrong! That first one was a killer! True, I didn't eat snacks as such, but I discovered that lots of food was reaching my mouth between meals. I did a lot of taste testing while I cooked. I ate leftovers instead of throwing them away. And I knew I was in big trouble when I realized that I was watching the kids and hoping they would stop eating soon, since anything left on their plates was fair game! You get the picture. I was eating the equivalent of a fourth meal every day! I can't tell you how difficult it was to change that one behavior. It takes most people three weeks to form a new habit. It took me every bit that long.

When at last the behavior that you have chosen begins to come more easily, add another until all of them are a part of your lifestyle. To do numbers three, four, and five you can enlist the help of a registered dietitian, or you can analyze your own diet. If you choose the do-it-yourself method, here's how to proceed. You'll need a pencil and a highlighter pen. Turn to the Fats of Life chart that begins on page 74 and follow these instructions:

1. Circle every food you eat four or more times per week. *Highlight* all circled foods in the medium, high, and "fat city" categories. (Check the labels of any package food you use for calories and grams of fat per serving.)
2. Next *circle* and *highlight* every food you eat four or more times per week that is high in sugar. (Some of these are low-fat but still high-calorie because sugar is a concentrated carbohydrate.) *Highlight* fruit but not vegetable juices.
3. If you drink alcohol, *circle* and *highlight* alcoholic drinks.

Now comes the hard part—deciding how to decrease your intake of the highlighted foods. Consider each food carefully. You have three options:

eat much less of that food,

or

substitute something from a low-fat category,

or

don't eat that food regularly.

Be realistic. You know yourself better than anyone else. Does one bite of Häagen-Dazs unleash an unquenchable desire for half a gallon? Then option three is the only possibility for that food. Trying number one would be absurd. For me, number two was a good choice in the case of mayonnaise. Low-calorie mayonnaise tastes good to me, so I never use regular mayonnaise now. Other fats can also be replaced with lower calorie counterparts—plain non- or low-fat yogurt for sour cream, low-calorie for regular salad dressings, etc.

Be creative. There are many ways to eat less of high-fat foods. Instead of pouring salad dressing on top, have it on the side and dip your fork into the dressing first and then into the salad. You'll use *much* less. Use half a pat of margarine instead of a whole one. Trim all the visible fat from meat. Remove the skin from chicken. Better yet, try pasta, legume, and other low-fat entrees in place of meat. Use low-fat or nonfat milk. With practice you will find many ways to cut calories by decreasing fat, and your tastes will change too. Now I can happily eat a baked potato with one-third the added margarine that I once used. The possibilities are endless. Find solutions you can live with. It's critical.

I lost about twenty-five pounds by following my own instructions up to this point. But to lose the last five tenacious pounds I had to haul out the heavy artillery—actually *counting* grams of fat and eating just twenty to forty grams per day. (Notice the grams of fat *per serving* at the top of each Fats of Life column.) A man could afford to eat thrity to sixty grams of fat per day. This regimen still permitted eating quite a lot of food, but *most* of it had to come from the "Hardly Any Fat" column and only *tiny* amounts from the "Fat City" column. It's tough, but it works. A pretty good rule of thumb is this: If you need to lose a lot of weight, restrict fat to twenty to forty grams per day if you're a woman, or thirty to sixty grams if you're a man, until you have lost 10 percent of your original weight. Then maintain this new weight for several months by following the general guidelines on page 70. That will give your body time to adjust its metabolic rate to defend the new, lower body weight. Now *count* grams of fat per day again until you lose 10 percent of your starting body weight, then maintain for a while again. Repeat the cycle as many times as necessary to reach your weight goal.

Now go back to the Fats of Life chart. Consider the circled foods that are *not* highlighted. Eat more of them. Look carefully at the "Hardly any fat" foods you didn't circle. Are there some you might enjoy that you don't eat now? Foods from this group can be used freely during meals. Many are high-fiber foods—fruits, vegetables, whole-grain products—that have the added benefit of making you feel full.

Now about number eleven—standing nude in front of a mirror every morning. You may think this one's ridiculous, but before you skip to the next paragraph, hear me out. Overweight people are notorious for rationalizing, "I'm not as fat as she is"; "it's really only a few pounds"; etc. I know, because I've used them all. Facing the bare facts sweeps those excuses away, and the memory of that double chin, those bulging hips, and the flabby thighs will help fortify you to withstand calorific temptations hours later. You don't need a lot of time. Getting dressed in front of a mirror is fine. That's what I do.

One other thing. There is a good way to speed up the process of building new habits. It's called "positive mental imaging." Athletes use it, and you can too. As an example, let's take my "fat habit" of eating while I did the dishes. After dinner my husband and I watch TV before I do the dishes. While we're watching TV, I can imagine myself going into the kitchen, picking up dishes, and scraping the food into the garbage disposer without putting anything into my mouth. The more graphic the picture, the better. I can do this several times during one commercial, and as far as my brain is concerned, *the result is the same as my actually doing it!* The new "skinny habit" is reinforced just as much as by "real" practice. Using this technique along with actual behavior change can greatly shorten the "practice" step.

Of course, there will be setbacks. Don't get discouraged when you regress to your old habits. Just keep recommitting yourself to the new lifestyle. Slowly but surely, the pounds will drop away. Your muscles will firm up, and your body will adjust to the new lower weight and defend against any deviation from it.

Capability

Becoming capable is the reward for the hard work of practice. Just as a piece of music that once seemed far beyond a musician's abilities can be played effortlessly after much practice, the new behaviors ultimately become easy. In fact they will become so natural that eventually it will be difficult for you to believe that you ever lived differently. Perhaps for the first time, you will feel in control of your life.

Positive attitude

With capability comes a positive attitude about the new lifestyle. Whereas at the practice stage you may have resented the necessary changes, now you will be positively evangelistic about your new behaviors. You will think everyone should adopt them! So a word of caution. Not all of your friends *want* to be converted. Although *you* know that life is infinitely richer and more meaningful now that you look and feel fantastic, not everyone is ready to change. Wait for the truly honest in heart to ask before you expound on your odyssey to fitness.

Motivation

The good feelings that you have about yourself make you *want* to continue the new behavior patterns. Now it's not so much a commitment as it is an addiction! You're "hooked" on something good.

Value

You have reached the highest step when the new behaviors are so important to you that you cherish them. When you reach this stage, your weight control will very likely be permanent. You cannot take all seven steps in a single bound. They require time and perseverance. But the results are priceless and lasting. Having experienced the rich rewards of fitness, life on any other plane will seem poor indeed.

---

1. Some medications for high blood pressure lower the maximum heart rate. If you are on high blood pressure medicine, ask your physician how your exercise program should be adjusted.

The Fats of Life

Bread & Cereal Group

Recommended Daily: 4 servings

Hardly Any Fat	Low Fat 30-40% calories as fat 5 gm fat/serving	Medium Fat 50% calories as fat 10 gm fat/serving	High Fat 60% calories as fat 15 gm fat/serving	Fat City 70% calories as fat 20 gm fat/serving
All cereals, cooked and dry, except granola Cornmeal Grits Pasta, spaghetti, macaroni, noodles, etc. Rice Bagels Breadsticks Yeast breads, all English muffins Pita bread Rolls Tortillas Crackers Crispbread-type Graham Matzo Melba toast Oyster crackers Popcorn (no butter) Pretzels Saltines Rice cakes Wheat germ	Arrowroot cookies, 6 Biscuit Bread stuffing, 1/4 c. Cornbread, 2" x 2" Chow mein noodles, 1/2 c. Granola cereal, 1 oz. Muffin Pancake, 5" diameter Party crackers (butter type), 10 Taco shells, 2 Tortilla chips, 1 oz. Waffle, 4" x 4"	Sweet rolls, 3" square Croissant	Cheese puffs, 1-1/2 oz. Corn chips, 1-1/2 oz.	

To find grams of fat and calories per serving, read labels.

To calculate percentage of calories as fat: $\dfrac{\text{gm fat/serving} \times 9}{\text{calories/serving}} \times 100$

The Fats of Life

Protein Group

Recommended Daily: Adult: Two 2 oz. serv. Child/Teen: Two serv. Pregnant: Three serv.

Hardly Any Fat	Low Fat 30-40% calories as fat 5 gm fat/serving	Medium Fat 50% calories as fat 10 gm fat/serving	High Fat 60% calories as fat 15 gm fat/serving	Fat City 70% calories as fat 20 gm fat/serving

Baked beans
1% cottage cheese
Dried beans and peas
Egg whites
Egg substitutes
without fat (read label)
Tuna, water pack
	Soybeans, ⅔ c.
	Cottage cheese,
	creamed 4%, ½ c.
	Diet cheese (less than
	55 calories/oz.) 2 oz.
		Beef, veal, lean (USDA
		Good or Choice), 3 oz.
		Chicken, without skin, 3 oz.
		Goat meat, 3-½ oz.
		Hamburger (10% fat by
		weight), 3 oz.
		Mozarella cheese
		(part skim), 2 oz.
		Parmesan cheese, 1 oz.
		Pork, lean, 3 oz.
		Tofu, 7 oz.
		Turkey, without skin, 3 oz.
			Beef roasts, 3 oz.
			Chicken with skin, 3 oz.
			Diet cheese (56-80
			calories/oz.), 2 oz.
			Eggs, 3
			Egg substitutes
			with fat, ¾ c.
			Hamburger (20% fat by
			weight), 3 oz.
			Lamb, chops, roast, 3 oz.
			Pork, loin, chops, 3 oz.
			Ricotta cheese, ½ c.
			Steak, 3 oz.
			Tuna, oil pack, ½ c.
				Bacon, 1-½ oz.
				Beef ribs, 2 oz.
				or 6 med. ribs
				Bologna, 2-½ oz.
				Duck, roasted with
				skin, 3 oz.
				Frankfurters, 2
				Goose, roasted with
				skin, 1-½ oz.
				Liverwurst, 2 oz.
				Peanut butter, 3 T.
				Salami, 2 oz.
				Sausage, 2 oz.
				Mozarella cheese, made
				with whole milk, 3 oz.
				Swiss cheese, 2 oz.
				Nuts:
				Half cup:
				  Cashews
				  Peanuts
				Third cup:
				  Almonds
				  Brazil nuts
				  Hazel nuts
				  Macadamia nuts
				  Pecans
				  Pistachios
				  Walnuts

To find grams of fat and calories per serving, read labels.

To calculate percentage of calories as fat: $\dfrac{\text{gm fat/serving} \times 9}{\text{calories/serving}} \times 100$

The Fats of Life

Milk Group

Recommended Daily:
Adult: Two serv.
Child: Three serv.
Teen: Four serv.
Pregnant: Four serv.

Hardly Any Fat	Low Fat 30–40% calories as fat 5 gm fat/serving	Medium Fat 50% calories as fat 10 gm fat/serving	High Fat 60% calories as fat 15 gm fat/serving	Fat City 70% calories as fat 20 gm fat/serving
1% milk Nonfat (skim) milk Buttermilk made from skim milk (cultured) Yogurt, nonfat	Buttermilk made from whole milk, 2 oz. 2% low-fat milk, 1 c. Yogurt, plain, made from 2% milk, 1 c. Custard, ⅓ c. Pudding, ½ c.	Diet cheese (56-80 calories/oz.), 2 oz. Whole milk (4% fat), 1 c. Evaporated milk (whole), ½ c. Yogurt, made from whole milk, 1 c. Diet cheese (less than 55 calories/oz.), 2 oz. Parmesan cheese, 1 oz. Mozzarella cheese (part skim), 2 oz. Ricotta cheese (part skim), ½ c.		American cheese, 2 oz. Cheddar cheese, 2 oz. Mozzarella cheese, made with whole milk, 3 oz. Ricotta cheese (whole), ⅔ c. Swiss cheese, 2 oz.

To find grams of fat and calories per serving, read labels.

To calculate percentage of calories as fat: $\dfrac{\text{gm fat/serving} \times 9}{\text{calories/serving}} \times 100$

The Fats of Life

Fruit & Vegetable Group — Recommended Daily: 4 servings

Hardly Any Fat	Low Fat 30-40% calories as fat 5 gm fat/serving	Medium Fat 50% calories as fat 10 gm fat/serving	High Fat 60% calories as fat 15 gm fat/serving	Fat City 70% calories as fat 20 gm fat/serving
All fruits and vegetables prepared without fat (except avocado—see Fat City) Fruit juices Vegetable juices	Soybeans, ⅔ c. Tortilla chips, 1 oz.	French fried potatoes, ½ c.	Potato chips, 1 oz. Corn chips, 1-½ oz.	Avocado, ½

To find grams of fat and calories per serving, read labels.

To calculate percentage of calories as fat: $\dfrac{\text{gm fat/serving} \times 9}{\text{calories/serving}} \times 100$

The Fats of Life

Extra Foods Group			None required: Limit intake		
Hardly Any Fat	Low Fat 30-40% calories as fat 5 gm fat/serving	Medium Fat 50% calories as fat 10 gm fat/serving	High Fat 60% calories as fat 15 gm fat/serving	Fat City 70% calories as fat 20 gm fat/serving

Alcoholic drinks
Angel food cake
Animal crackers
Fig bar cookies
Fudgesicle
Ices
Jelly
Soft drinks
Syrup
Sugar
Hard candy
	Arrowroot cookies, 6
	Cookies, sugar,
	  oatmeal, butter, 2 med.
	Fudge, with nuts, 1 oz.
	Gingerbread, 1 piece
	Granola bar
	Ice cream sandwich
	Vanilla wafers, 7
	Pie, fruit, $\frac{1}{16}$ of pie
		Cake, iced, 1 piece
		Cookies, chocolate chip, 3
		Doughnut, 3-$\frac{1}{2}$"
		Ice cream (10% fat), $\frac{2}{3}$ c.
			Chocolate candy bar, $\frac{1}{2}$ oz.
			Ice cream, rich
			  (16% fat), $\frac{2}{3}$ c.
				Butter, 5 t.
				Chocolate-covered
				  nuts, 1-$\frac{1}{2}$ oz.
				Cream cheese, $\frac{1}{4}$ c.
				Eclair with whipped cream
				Lard, 5 t.
				Margarine, 5 t.
				Mayonnaise, 5 t.
				Oils, 5 t.
				Sour cream, $\frac{1}{2}$ c.
				Cream, light, $\frac{1}{3}$ c.
				Salad dressing, 3 T.
				Whipping cream, $\frac{1}{4}$ c.

To find grams of fat and calories per serving, read labels.

To calculate percentage of calories as fat: $\dfrac{\text{gm fat/serving} \times 9}{\text{calories/serving}} \times 100$

Chapter 10

When thin is not in

Several years ago I had a student whose name was Rey. It suited him perfectly. Like a wood-burning stove on a winter's day, he fairly radiated warmth and energy. Not every topic we studied captured his imagination, but the subject of anorexia nervosa fascinated him. Rey began caring for a young anorexic woman as part of his clinical experience as a student dietitian. I never saw the patient myself, but I grew to feel that I knew her as Rey excitedly reported on her progress. It was beautiful to see Rey's enthusiasm. And I was glad for the positive outcome, not only for the patient's sake, but also for the encouragement that it gave to Rey.

Months passed, and with the springtime came commencement day. Rey graduated and moved to Europe, and I did not think of his patient again until the next autumn when I lectured on anorexia to the new class of students. It was then that I learned she had died of starvation. I was stunned.

Little scraps of conversation with Rey flitted through my mind. I remembered that his patient was from an affluent home, highly intelligent, a graduate student pursuing a master's degree. And now all the bright hopes that she and her parents had had for the future were snuffed out.

I tell this story for two reasons. First, because I hope it will push aside the façade of superficiality that eating disorders often wear and expose them for what they really are—potentially lethal conditions. And second, I want to suggest that in this realm there are no quick fixes.

It has been said, "You can never be too rich or too thin." I can't be sure about the rich part, but I know for certain that you can be too thin. Anyone who can count every rib just by looking is too thin. Reducing your percent of body fat so low that menstruation ceases is too thin. Depriving your body of calories so that it is forced to break down its own tissue with resulting death from heart failure is too thin. Yet each of these situations is familiar to professionals dealing with victims of eating disorders. And their numbers are growing. It is estimated that up to one-third of women students at some American colleges are suffering from some type of eating disorder, and men are also being affected in increasing numbers.

Probably the best known of the eating disorders is anorexia nervosa. Singer Karen Carpenter's death in 1983 served to focus national attention on this condition. But several other eating disorders are very common in this country. The other leading contenders are bulimia and compulsive overeating. All three can be fatal. Aside from that fact, they appear to be very dissimilar on the surface, but a deeper look reveals many similarities. Three women—Jan, Laura, and Michelle—are typical examples of these three eating disorders.

Jan

Jan had everything. It was hard not to stare as she leaned against the mast of the sailboat as it skimmed across the sparkling water. Her golden mass of long hair rippled in the breeze and caught the sunlight, making it shine as if it were on fire. Her laughing blue eyes made her classic features come alive. But most of all, her voluptuous body riveted your eye.

It never even crossed my mind that this college freshman was the victim of an eating disorder. But she was. Bulimia. Jan grew up in a world of "beautiful people." Her father was a successful surgeon, and her mother also had a career. They lived in a Spanish-style house. Appearances were important. Jan's mother had a tendency toward plumpness and always seemed to be on a diet. As Jan matured, she was distressed to find that her body didn't match the slim shapes of the models in the fashion magazines.

And she loved to eat, especially when the stress was really bad at school or her love life was disappointing. Drowning her sorrows in sweet, gooey food really helped—except when her weight soared. Then Jan felt even worse.

But a "wonderful" thing happened. Jan discovered purging. Why hadn't she thought of this before? She could eat enormous amounts of anything—ice cream, chips and dip, cookies, brownies—and then vomit it all up. By the time she was a freshman in college, Jan had developed the typical binge/purge cycle. She was vomiting several times a day. It got easier all the time. Whereas in the beginning she needed to stick a spoon handle down her throat to induce vomiting, now a light tickle with a fingernail did the trick. The stresses of college life drove her more and more to the sweet relief of bingeing. She left the campus more committed to the binge/purge cycle than when she came.

Many aspects of Jan's story are typical of bulimia. Outwardly, the victim often displays no obvious clue that anything is wrong. Not only is her weight normal,[1] she may even be slightly overweight. Unlike the anorexic, she feels ashamed about her behavior and tries to hide the vomiting and abuse of laxatives and diuretics from her family and friends. Looks are all important. In fact, her entire self-image seems to hinge on being physically attractive, especially to men. Sexual promiscuity, as well as lying and stealing, are fairly common. Food provides a comforting emotional anesthetic, much like the effect of alcohol on an alcoholic. And it can be just as addicting.

One victim of bulimia told me that she felt forced to stop and purchase food at every possible opportunity as she drove. It wasn't so much a conscious choice as it was a compulsion.

During a binge the bulimic may consume as many as 1,000 to 10,000 calories, followed by feelings of overwhelming guilt, with subsequent vomiting and/or purging with laxatives and diuretics and often sleep. The chosen foods are usually high in carbohydrate and fat, such as doughnuts, cake, cookies, peanut butter,

---

1. While the majority of bulimics are women, some men do have the problem.

etc., and do not require much chewing. In the beginning the victim doesn't dream that she is starting down the road to an obsession in which the anxiety/relief/guilt cycle will progressively take over her life, and that it will drive her to ever more intense and frequent bingeing episodes followed by purging, guilt, and depression, which in turn demand relief through eating. The comforting "solution" of bingeing produces the very fear and depression it was intended to relieve. This cycle ultimately dominates the victim's life, robbing her of any real satisfaction or peace.

Bulimic episodes may continue for quite some time before any physical symptoms appear. The first of these is often a chronically sore throat and heartburn. Later, erosion of the teeth from frequent exposure to digestive fluids is often seen. Some girls have had to have all their teeth capped as a result. If there is no intervention, electrolyte (mineral) imbalance can result in cardiac arrest, causing death.

Laura

Laura was obviously very sick. When she finally sought professional help, she weighed seventy-eight pounds, even though she was five feet, five inches tall. Her skin stretched tautly over the sharp bones of her hips, and every contour of her ribs and spine were painfully obvious.

Though just a teenager, Laura's eating disorder was not new. It was hard to say when she began limiting the amount she allowed herself to eat. At first she just wanted to lose a few pounds. When she succeeded, the euphoria and sense of control spurred her to lose more. Again she experienced success and a sense of power. She couldn't remember ever feeling so good. Before this she had always felt trapped and unable to control anything in her life.

Laura's parents had decided to divorce when she was three, but they didn't actually do so until she was thirteen! During those ten years, Laura unconsciously did many things to focus her parents' attention on her and away from the problems between themselves. She desperately tried to please them and make them proud of her. And they had such high expectations!

How Laura should look and behave and perform in school were all clearly outlined for her. Before she started dieting, Laura couldn't remember ever having set and achieved a goal of her own. Her whole life had been planned for her.

Even though she progressively began to starve herself, Laura became an excellent cook. She delighted in preparing wonderful meals for her parents and sister. She herself ate little or nothing, and eventually she no longer ate with the family. She preferred to eat alone in her room. There no one commented on the minute portions she took or the fact that she cut the food into tiny pieces, chewed a mouthful, and then spit it out into a napkin. It was amazing how much time she could spend eating practically nothing. Yet in spite of her microscopic energy intake, her output was tremendous. She exercised compulsively, never letting a day go by without vigorous physical activity that would have been astonishing even in a well-nourished athlete.

Laura's story graphically illustrates the issue underlying most cases of anorexia nervosa—*control*. In her case, the family played a major role. This is often true, but the family can also be a wonderful ally in helping the anorexic resolve the emotional issues driving her to engage in disordered eating behavior. In fact, if the anorexic is young and living at home, recovery is doubtful *unless* the family becomes involved with her in therapeutic counseling. And recovery is possible. The process will be long and sometimes painful, but the alternative may be the victim's death, or at best, a life bereft of hope and filled with depression and despair.

Michelle

Michelle was chubby even as a baby, and by the time she reached puberty her five-foot-four-inch frame supported over two hundred pounds. When I first met her, she was thirty-two and weighed 330 pounds. Just walking was an effort, and I noticed that she was adept at using her children to perform routine tasks for her. She had constant physical problems ranging from heartburn and hypoglycemia to lumps in her breasts. Like her body, Michelle's medical chart was thick and growing.

It was not surprising that Michelle became overweight. Both her parents tended toward obesity. Michelle herself absolutely loved food. She loved buying it. She loved cooking it. And she especially loved eating it.

Boys didn't flock to Michelle as they did to some of her friends, and eating took away some of the pain. More than anything, she wanted a permanent boyfriend. But relationships never worked out the way she expected, and each disappointment diminished her self-esteem a little more. But food never failed her.

Michelle was typical of many compulsive overeaters. She literally could not control herself when it came to food. If she ate one slice of cake, she couldn't help finishing off the whole thing. The drive to eat went far beyond the mere relief of hunger. It was motivated by an intense longing to fill a void, a great emptiness within. An obese patient described this phenomenon best when she told me, "It's eating to satisfy a hunger that cannot be satisfied."

When I first saw her, Michelle was already experiencing some obesity-related health problems. Compulsive overeaters are at risk of developing high blood pressure. Since the heart must supply all body tissues with blood, the extra pounds make it work much harder. The joints are often damaged from carrying excess weight. Gallstones are common, and the risk of surgical complications is higher because anesthetics are fat soluble. Blood cholesterol levels often rise, and susceptible persons may develop type II diabetes. Certain cancers are more common to the overweight. Death certificates of compulsive overeaters often list heart attack or stroke as the cause of death.

Danger signs

Since eating disorders are serious, it is important that they be treated. Even though anorexia, bulimia, and compulsive overeating are each unique problems, they have certain common warning signs. In each there will be:

- an unhealthy amount of body fat (too much or too little),

- abnormal attitudes and behavior toward food.

A gross assessment called Body Mass Index (BMI) will indicate whether body fat is a problem. To find your BMI, draw a straight line on the chart below from your weight in pounds on the left to your height in inches on the right. Mark the line in the center where the straight edge crosses it. This is your BMI.

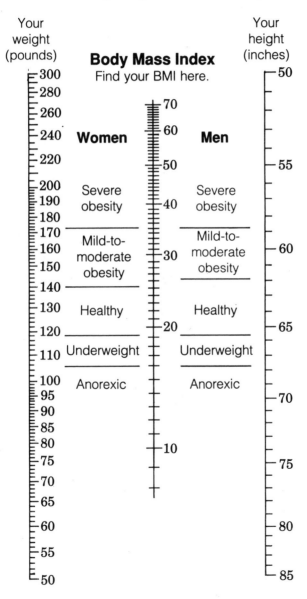

Your weight (pounds)

Body Mass Index
Find your BMI here.

Your height (inches)

Women

Men

Severe obesity

Severe obesity

Mild-to-moderate obesity

Mild-to-moderate obesity

Healthy

Healthy

Underweight

Underweight

Anorexic

Anorexic

In general, BMIs indicate the following:

Healthy	BMI 19 to 26
Underweight	BMI 16 to 19
Anorexic	BMI 18 or under
Bulimic	BMI 16 to 19 or up to 26 (varies)
Overweight	BMI 26 to 35
Severe obesity	BMI 35 or above

The Body Mass Index will provide a clue indicating anorexia or compulsive overeating. Bulimia is harder to pinpoint, but noticeable fluctuations in weight are a red flag. In diagnosing all three disorders it is important to look at eating behaviors. Is the person *preoccupied* with body weight and/or the buying and preparing of food? What about the location, timing, size of servings, and eating behavior at meals? Does one of the eating disorder charts include many characteristics you have observed? One or two symptoms are not a cause for alarm, but if one-third to one-half of the listed characteristics are present, it is likely that a problem exists.

What to do

Each person is unique, and what works for one may not for another. *Recovery is possible*, but there are two essentials: a health professional who is skilled in treating eating disorders, and the patient's commitment to recovery.

Anorexia. Treatment of anorexia may be either as an outpatient or inpatient. Hospitalization *may* be necessary if the patient has lost up to 30 percent of her original weight, and it will be *essential* if weight loss has become life threatening. Therefore, the first goal during hospitalization is to promote weight gain. Hopefully this can be done through eating regular food, but in the most severe cases it is necessary to feed the patient by tube or by vein in order to save his/her life. As the patient begins to regain weight (and usually not before) she is able to profit from counseling.

Eating disorder treatment centers take a variety of approaches, but psychological counseling is included in virtually all of them, and it is the major focus of many programs. This counseling can take several forms, including individual, group, and family. Each can be valuable at different stages of recovery. Drug therapy (antidepressants) may also be used. For more information about anorexia, contact one of the following organizations:

American Anorexia/Bulimia Assoc., Inc.
418 E. 76th St.
New York, NY 10021
Phone: 212-734-1114

National Anorectic Aid Society
1925 Dublin-Granville Rd.
Columbus, Ohio 43229
Phone: 614-436-1112

Bulimia. It is usually impossible for a bulimic to break the binge/purge cycle alone. Most victims need psychological counseling, and perhaps drug therapy. One theory holds that underlying bulimia is a biologically caused depression that antidepressant medications may help to relieve. Group therapy is often extremely valuable. To get help, consult a psychiatrist, psychologist, or eating disorder unit.

Compulsive overeating. Treatment ranges from behavior modification to starvation diets, drugs, and drastic surgery that permanently limits food intake. I urge that behavior modification be tried first. This is discussed in the chapter, "Permanent girth control." Before beginning, enlist the support of family and friends. Get someone to exercise with you and to encourage you in the practice of new food habits.

Joining an organized support group such as Overeaters Anonymous, Weight Watchers, or TOPS can help enormously. The emotional support is invaluable.

If these strategies fail, you should consider more drastic measures. Very low calorie diets (under 1,000 calories per day) are effective, but they *must* be monitored by a physician. As noted in the chapter on girth control, such diets are not without hazards, some of which are life threatening. Therefore, the very low calorie diets are justified only if you must lose more than fifty pounds.

The use of drugs in the treatment of overweight can be effective, but it may have side effects such as high blood pressure, insomnia, and digestive disturbances. Many drugs are also habit forming. Also, many people regain lost weight when the drugs are discontinued. For these reasons I feel that it is best to avoid using drugs for weight control.

Surgery is a last-ditch strategy to achieve weight loss. Many surgical procedures are currently in use. Fat cells can actually be sucked out by a process called "liposuction." All the hazards of surgery are present, of course, and following surgery, new fat cells will be formed if more calories are eaten than are used. Therefore, a change in eating and exercising habits is important following liposuction.

In gastric stapling a double row of staples across the stomach makes a tiny food pouch that only holds about two ounces. Vomiting occurs if more than two ounces are eaten. Because food intake is drastically reduced, the loss in weight is usually dramatic. Some patients successfully maintain this weight loss, but many regain slowly, beginning one to three years following the surgery, probably due to stretching of the pouch.

In an operation similar to gastric stapling, an inflated balloon is left in the stomach, which produces results much like those following gastric stapling. Wiring the jaws shut is another surgical procedure producing good short-term results. However, none of the drastic surgeries should be considered unless you need to lose a great deal of weight, usually 100 pounds or more, and only after you have tried less-drastic weight control measures first.

Back to Jan, Laura, and Michelle

The stories of Jan, Laura, and Michelle illustrated well the typical characteristics of bulimia, anorexia, and compulsive overeating. Their ultimate fates also demonstrate the gamut from failure to success that therapists achieve with eating disorder patients.

I often wonder whether Jan ever reached the point of seeking help, because during her years at college she never did. She cherished her binge/purge behavior so much that she was blinded to its seriousness. She even encouraged others to use the bulimic method of weight control. This denial of the problem is common and extremely difficult to combat. One patient here at Loma Linda University Medical Center was shocked into facing reality only after another member of her therapy group suddenly died. Fortunately, skillful therapists are often able to break through the denial. This step is essential before healing can begin, and as far as I know, Jan never took it. I hope that the inevitable minor physical problems caused by bulimia will drive her to seek help before a medical emergency threatens her very life.

Laura's story had a happier ending. She was extremely wasted when she finally began treatment—a situation that does not bode well for the future. In fact, the earlier anorexia nervosa is treated, the better the chances are for a complete recovery. But Laura was one of the lucky ones. Even though her disorder had reduced her to a virtual skeleton, skillful treatment slowly clothed her body in healthy flesh and her mind with rational thought. In her twenties now, Laura is supporting herself and living on her own.

I recently saw Michelle. She looks very different from the 330-pound woman I first met several years ago. Losing over 100 pounds has made a tremendous difference not only in her looks but also in her life. It has boosted her self-image, and this has enabled her to advance professionally to a position so challenging that the buying, preparing, and eating of food is no longer central to her existence. I'm happy to say that she accomplished this weight loss solely through changing her eating and exercising habits. It took time, but the results have lasted. In Michelle's case, Overeaters Anonymous, with its twelve-step program, supported this lifestyle change. Most compulsive overeaters need a support group if they are to be successful in the long run, and I highly recommend finding one.

If you see yourself in Jan, Laura, or Michelle, do yourself a favor. Get help. Because you're worth it.

Bulimia

Low self-esteem
Usually female between seventeen and twenty-five years of age
Self-worth dependent on being thin
Weight fluctuations—may be below, at, or slightly above normal
Obsession with body image and weight
Self-induced vomiting
Abuse of laxatives
Abuse of diuretics
Develops binge/purge cycle
Poor impulse control
Ashamed of bulimic behavior
Anxious
Depressed
Eats alone
Preoccupied with food and eating
Tired
Apathetic
Irritable
Gastrointestinal disorders
Withdraws from normal activities
Distances self from family and friends
Lies
Steals (food, money, laxatives, diuretics)
Eroded teeth
Gum disease
Drug and alcohol abuse
Mood swings
Chronic sore throat
Difficulty swallowing and breathing
Constant physical problems, general poor health
Hypokalemia (abnormally low levels of potassium in the blood)
Electrolyte imbalance
Dehydration
Irregular heartbeat
Rupture of the esophagus/stomach
Suicide attempts

Anorexia nervosa

Low self-esteem
Usually female between twelve and thirty years of age
Feels lack of control over own life

Distorted body image (sees self as being fat when actually thin)
Overachiever
Compliant
Anxious
Cessation of menstruation
Abnormal eating patterns (i.e, chewing but not swallowing, cutting
    food into tiny pieces)
Precise counting of calories and extreme calorie restriction
Preoccupation with food and its preparation
Self-imposed isolation from family and friends
Perfectionistic
Compulsive exercising
Eats alone
Feels great satisfaction with progressive weight loss
Fights with family
Enlarged salivary glands (chipmunk cheeks)
Thinning hair on scalp
Increased fine facial and body hair
Skin of scalp is dry and thin
Marked weight loss (at least 20 percent of former weight)
Rigid
Depressed
Apathetic
Fear of food and of fatness
Malnourished
Manipulative
Mood swings (tyrannical)
Difficulty thinking
Cold
Weakness due to electrolyte (mineral) imbalance
Denial of problem
Sleep disturbances
Joint pain

Compulsive overeating

Low self-esteem
Both sexes affected, though more common in women
Weight exceeds 20 percent above ideal body weight
Rapid eating, taking large bites
May eat without feeling pleasure
Preoccupied with the buying, preparing, and eating of food
Little physical activity

Shortness of breath with mild exertion
Often socially isolated
Sleep apnea (breathing stops temporarily during sleep)
Binge eating, perhaps even after a large meal
Anger when confronted about body weight
Multiple unsuccessful attempts at weight control
Loss of control over food while eating
High blood pressure
High blood cholesterol level

Chapter 11

Soul food

The music of the lovely words made me read and reread them several times when I first encountered James Terry White's poem "Not by Bread Alone."

> If thou of fortune be bereft
> And in thy store there be but left
> Two loaves—sell one, and with the dole
> Buy hyacinths to feed thy soul.

I closed my eyes and said the lines over and over until I remembered them perfectly. And I knew exactly what they meant. Souls get hungry too.

Like every child, I often felt the hungering of the spirit, but I thought then that feeding the soul was an option. It would be many years before I knew that feeding the body without feeding the soul can never bring optimal health. It took time to learn that the body and the mind are inextricably linked, and that failing to nurture one is always sadly reflected in the other. I needed to see how holding a premature baby while it was being fed produced more weight gain than leaving it in an incubator and giving the same formula through a feeding tube. I needed to listen to a bulimic teenager describe her obsession to gorge on food when stressed. And most of all, I needed to watch my own children as they grew.

I wish I could say that I have learned all the "nutrients" necessary to build a strong and lovely spirit in a healthy body, but the truth is that I'm still learning every day. There are, however, three basics that I now believe to be vital.

Being there

Our children ate almost all their meals at the table, and when they were very young I noticed something interesting. As long as I was in the room and kept the conversational ball rolling, all three children ate well. But if I left for even a few minutes, nobody was eating when I got back. Often they had gotten up and were milling around the room! Many adults would rather not eat at all than to eat alone. Some lonely people react by *over*eating, but the underlying hunger for companionship is the same in either case.

But just being present physically is not enough. My friend Brett can testify to that. Her father made every meal of her childhood so painful by his critical, derogatory remarks that even now, thirty years later, Brett actually finds it hard to sit down at a dinner table. She usually eats standing up.

So even though I'm quite sure that being there physically is important, I'm even more sure that being there *emotionally* is what truly feeds the soul. Empathy has great power to nourish and heal. Communicating it is a priceless gift, and I think it is often packaged in a receptive gaze, a tone of voice, laughter, open body language, or active listening.

Beauty

Everybody knows that we eat with our eyes, but living in the fast lane leaves most of us little time for setting a beautiful table. I decided to at least make dinner on Friday night special. The food was simplicity itself—chili, fresh-baked bread (made from frozen dough), fruit salad, milk, dessert—but the setting was attractive. We ate in the dining room by candlelight and used the best china, silver, and crystal. I chose Friday night because our family is Seventh-day Adventist, and for us sundown marks the beginning of the Sabbath. For me, it was an oasis, a pool of calm where the five of us renewed our spirits.

Yet I often wondered if the children even cared. The boys seemed more interested in blowing out the candles. Then one day my husband got home at four, having skipped lunch, so I fed him immediately. At six o'clock Stephanie and Steve were nowhere to be seen, but eight-year-old Scott was hungry, so I sat him down to a plate of food in the kitchen. He sat motionless for several seconds, then looked up and asked, "No candles? This silver? This is Friday night, isn't it?"

The next week we all ate together in the dining room!

Acceptance

Like people everywhere, I always accept and love my family and friends. Whether or not we agree and share the same values, my affection for them remains unchanged. *Really.* Unfortunately, this is not how I always come across.

Stephen was terribly slow about getting dressed for kindergarten one day. Since he was engrossed in the story he was telling, I slipped a handsome new shirt over his head and hoped he wouldn't notice. I should have known better. One glance down and he exploded. "I won't wear this shirt! I don't like it!" He raced up the stairs, reappearing a moment later with his favorite old sweatshirt. I was proud that during the ensuing altercation I never raised my voice once and accepted defeat rather gracefully. I kissed him goodbye and watched as he walked down the driveway. But I was surprised to see him suddenly stop, turn, and start back toward the house. He confronted me at the door and said, "I won't go till you talk nice to me."

While it is true that I had never loved him more than when he refused to wear the new shirt, my reaction had made him feel rejected. I had robbed him of "soul food," which he needed so much that he was unwilling to go without it for even three hours. I'm glad that he came back and gave me a second chance. But how many other times have I done something similar to people without even recognizing it? I know now that the damage done is as serious as withholding bodily food.

Each spring the hyacinths remind me of White's poem. Souls do get hungry, and their feeding is not a whimsical option to be seized or dropped at will, but an obligation as real as nourishing the body. Because we do not live by bread alone.

Good health never tasted so good!

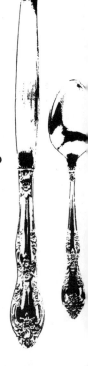

Life's Simple Pleasures redefines good eating and good times by providing complete seasonal menus (more than 140 mouthwatering, low-cholesterol, vegetarian recipes) that are easy to prepare and perfect for entertaining.

Spectacular color photographs stimulate the imagination of the creative host or hostess, returning joy to the kitchen and excitement to the dining table.

An excellent gift idea, *Life's Simple Pleasures* is more than a cookbook. It's a celebration of the good life.

US$24.95/Cdn$31.20. Hardcover, 160 pages.

Please photocopy and complete
the form below.

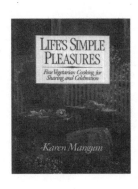